# Assessment of the Lower Limb

*For Churchill Livingstone:*

*Publishing Director, Health Professions:* Mary Law
*Project Development Manager:* Claire Wilson
*Project Manager:* Derek Robertson
*Design Direction:* Judith Wright

# Acknowledgements

We are indebted to those who have given their help and encouragement throughout the development and production of this second edition: in particular, our family and friends.

A big thank you to all the contributors for their time and effort in updating and/or rewriting their chapters. We would also like to thank Ann Marie Carr for her help with the new chapter on assessment of the elderly.

This book is dedicated to Jackie McLeod Roberts in recognition of her contribution to podiatry and in particular her work in the Ukraine, developing and improving footcare services for people with diabetes. Jackie's pioneering work has made a significant difference to these people.

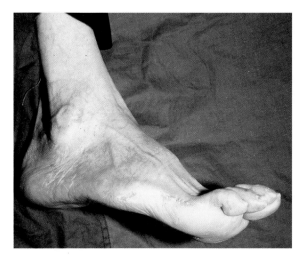

**Plate 1** An ischaemic foot. The superficial tissues are atrophied. The fifth ray has been excised.

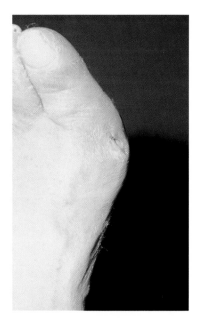

**Plate 2**
Typical ischaemic ulceration overlying a hallux abductovalgus in a patient with chronic peripheral vascular disease.

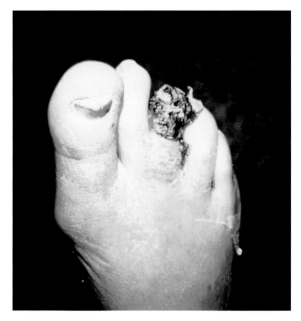

**Plate 3** 'Dry' gangrene, involving two toes. The necrotic area is surrounded by a narrow band of inflammation. The toes have become mummified, due to loss of the local blood supply.

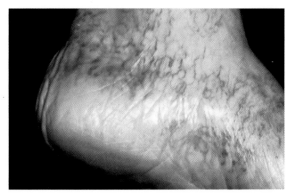

**Plate 4** Telangiectasias: distortion of the superficial venules secondary to varicosity.

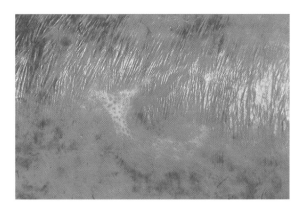

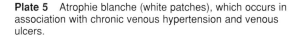

**Plate 5** Atrophie blanche (white patches), which occurs in association with chronic venous hypertension and venous ulcers.

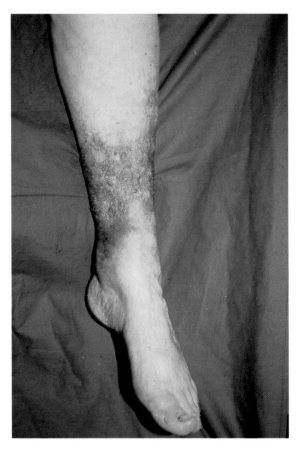

**Plate 6** Gravitational (varicose, stasis) eczema and haemosiderosis.

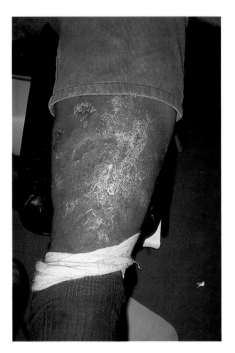

**Plate 7** Healed venous ulcer that had been present for 2 years.

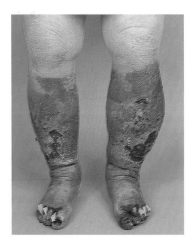

**Plate 8** Venous ulceration in association with gross oedema and haemosiderosis (from Wilkinson J, Shaw S, Fenton D 1993 Colour guide to dermatology. Churchill Livingstone, Edinburgh, Figure 179).

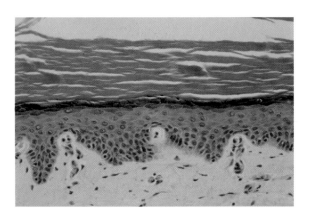

**Plate 9** Histology section of normal hairy skin stained with haematoxylin and eosin. Light microscopy × 60.

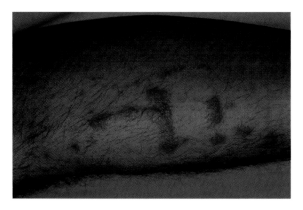

**Plate 10**  Koebner phenomenon in psoriasis due to injury.

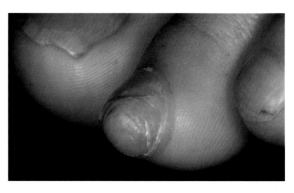

**Plate 11**  Subungual exostosis affecting the second toe.

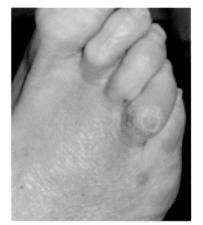

**Plate 13**
Dorsal corn.

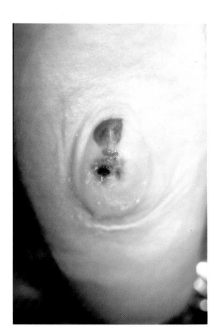

**Plate 12**
Extravasation within callus due to prolonged high pressure.

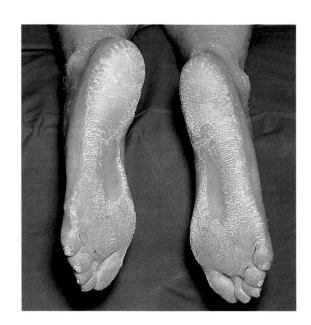

**Plate 14**  Plantar keratoderma.

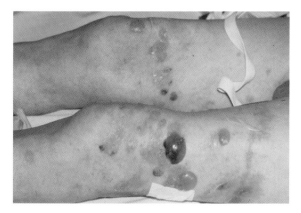

**Plate 15** Bullous pemphigoid.

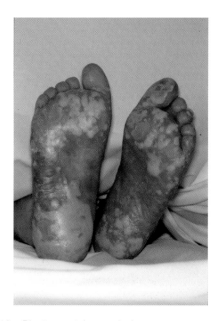

**Plate 16** Plantar pustular psoriasis.

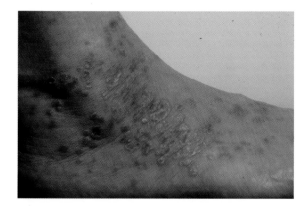

**Plate 17** Lichen planus.

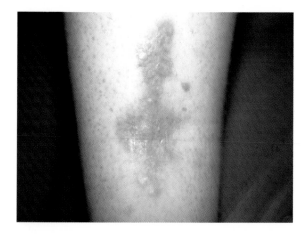

**Plate 18** Necrobiosis lipoidica.

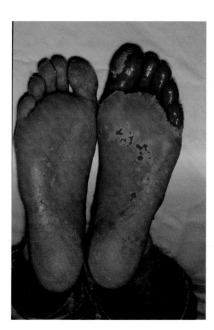

**Plate 19** Acute contact dermatitis to adhesives in footwear.

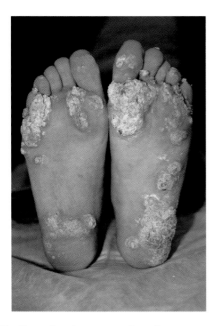

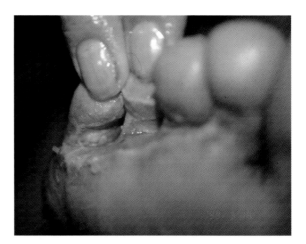

**Plate 21**   Pseudomonas infection affecting the interdigital area.

**Plate 20**   Extensive plantar warts in an immunosuppressed patient.

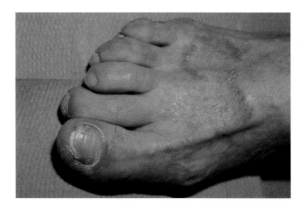

**Plate 23**   Tinea pedis affecting the dorsum of the foot.

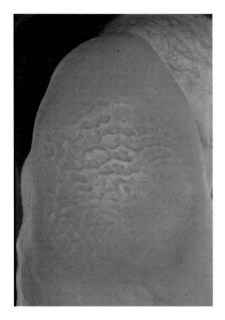

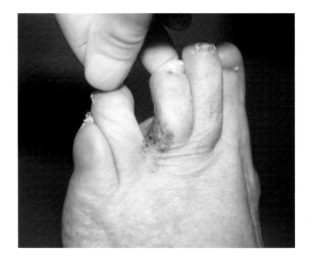

**Plate 22**   Pitted keratolysis of the heel.

**Plate 24**   Interdigital melanoma.

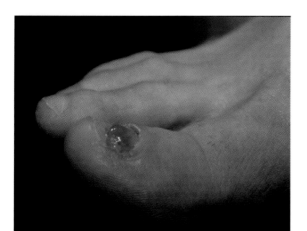

**Plate 25** Pyogenic granuloma under the nail.

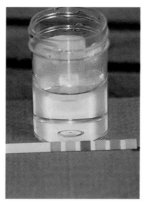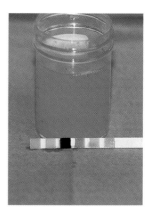

**Plate 27** The sample of urine on the left is normal; the sample on the right is cloudy and tinged with blood, indicating infection.

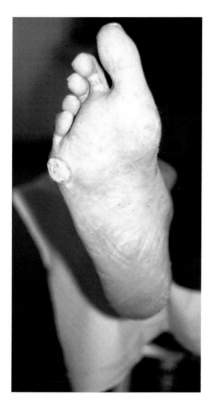

**Plate 26** Metastatic lesion (secondary from a lung tumour).

Bayer Diagnostics

ames

*Multistix* ®
**8SG**

New Formula

**Reagent Strips for Urinalysis** *For In Vitro Diagnostic Use*
Glucose, Ketone, Specific Gravity, Blood, pH, Protein, Nitrite, Leucocytes

PRINT DATE: 02/92     DO NOT USE AFTER: 02/94
DO NOT EXPOSE TO DIRECT SUNLIGHT
READ PRODUCT INSERT BEFORE USE.

**TESTS AND READING TIMES** (to be read in the direction of arrow)

| | | | | | | |
|---|---|---|---|---|---|---|
| **LEUCOCYTES** 2 minutes | NEG. | | TRACE | SMALL + | MODERATE ++ | LARGE +++ |
| **NITRITE** 60 seconds | NEG. | | | POSITIVE (any degree of uniform pink colour) | | |
| **PROTEIN** 60 seconds | NEG. | g/L TRACE | 0.30 + | 1 ++ | 3 +++ | ≥ 20 ++++ |
| **pH** 60 seconds | 5.0 | 6.0 | 6.5 | 7.0 | 7.5 | 8.0 | 8.5 |
| **BLOOD** 60 seconds | NEG. | NON-HAEMOLYZED TRACE | HAEMOLYZED TRACE | SMALL + | MODERATE ++ | LARGE +++ |
| **SPECIFIC GRAVITY** 45 seconds | 1.000 | 1.005 | 1.010 | 1.015 | 1.020 | 1.025 | 1.030 |
| **KETONE** 40 seconds | NEG. | mmol/L | TRACE 0.5 | SMALL 1.5 | MODERATE 4 | LARGE 8 | 16 |
| **GLUCOSE** 30 seconds | NEG. | mmol/L | 5.5 TRACE | 14 + | 28 ++ | 55 +++ | ≥111 ++++ |
| HANDLE END | | | | | | |

BR1600/H ENGLISH 11/91 Manufactured in UK

Bayer Diagnostics UK Limited Evans House, Hamilton Close, Basingstoke, Hampshire RG21 2YE

Multistix is a Trademark of Miles Inc. USA

**Plate 28** Multistix 8SG: the range of biochemical tests available from one urine sample (reproduced by kind permission of Bayer Diagnostics UK Ltd).

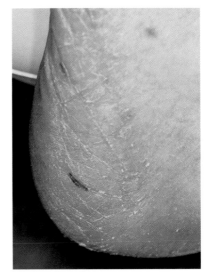

**Plate 29** Dry fissures develop when the skin is too brittle to conform to external and internal mechanical stresses (tension and shear particularly). They are a frequent complication of anhidrosis and atrophy.

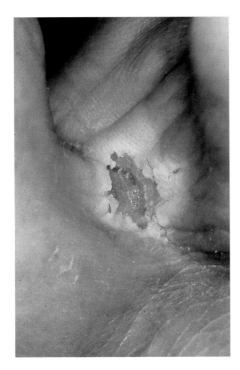

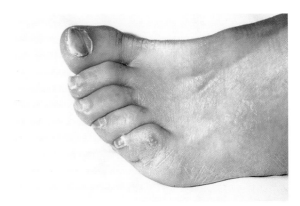

**Plate 31**   A typical neuropathic foot.

**Plate 30**   Hyperhidrosis, particularly interdigitally, leads to over-moist skin (macerated) which tears easily when mechanically stressed, sometimes exposing the dermis as seen here. Complications of hyperhidrosis include dermatophyte, yeast and bacterial infections.

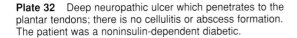

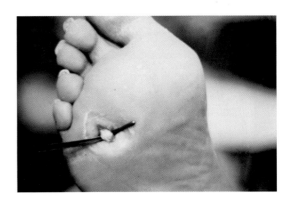

**Plate 32**   Deep neuropathic ulcer which penetrates to the plantar tendons; there is no cellulitis or abscess formation. The patient was a noninsulin-dependent diabetic.

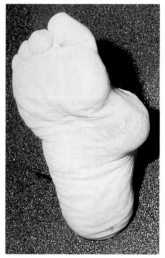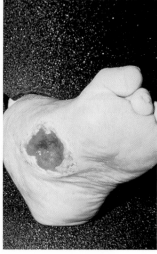

**Plate 33**  Bilateral arthropathy of the midtarsal joint, with ulceration of normally non-weightbearing soft tissues, in an insulin-dependent diabetic with peripheral neuropathy.

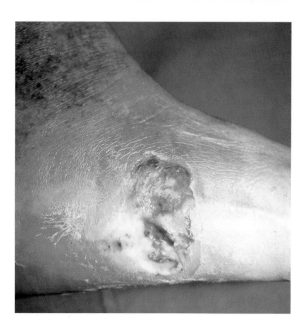

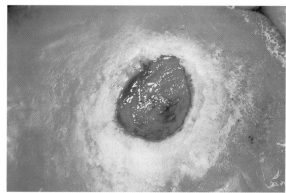

**Plate 34**  A neuropathic ulcer on the plantar surface of the foot.

**Plate 35**  Typical neuroischaemic ulceration over the lateral aspect of the midfoot in a noninsulin-dependent diabetic, showing deep erosion of soft tissues, sloughy base, heavy peripheral callosity and maceration of superficial tissues.

# Approaching the patient

# 1

# Assessment

*L. Merriman*

---

## INTRODUCTION

Patients present with a range of signs and symptoms for which they are seeking relief and if possible a cure. However, before this can be achieved, it is essential to undertake a primary patient assessment. Ineffective and inappropriate treatment may result if the practitioner has not taken into account information obtained from the assessment. This chapter explores why it is necessary to undertake an assessment and considers specific aspects of the assessment process.

## Why undertake a primary patient assessment?

Information from the assessment helps the practitioner to:

- arrive at a differential diagnosis or definitive diagnosis
- identify the likely cause of the problem (aetiology), e.g. trauma, pathogenic microorganism
- identify any factors which may influence the choice of treatment, e.g. poor blood supply, current drug regimen
- assess the extent of pathological changes so that a prognosis can be made
- establish a baseline in order to identify whether the condition is deteriorating or improving
- assess whether a second opinion is necessary.

All the above information is essential if the practitioner is to provide effective treatment and care for the patient.

## THE ASSESSMENT PROCESS

Assessment comprises three elements; the interview, observation and tests (Table 1.1). Information from the interview and observation is used to formulate ideas as to the likely diagnosis and cause. Further information may be sought via the interview and the use of clinical and laboratory tests. The practitioner uses the data gained from the assessment to formulate a hypothesis(es) from which a diagnosis will be reached. This diagnosis will be used to inform the management plan (Fig. 1.1). Where possible, the cause (aetiology) of the problem should be identified, as part of the management plan would be to eradicate or reduce the effects of the cause.

What has been outlined above is the ideal. In reality, patients often present with ill-defined problems and it is not possible to reach a definitive diagnosis. In these instances the practitioner explores a range of likely possibilities and develops the management plan in relation to these

**Table 1.1** Components of an assessment

| Component | |
| --- | --- |
| Assessment interview | Presenting problem |
| | Personal details |
| | Medical history |
| | Family history |
| | Social history |
| | Current health status |
| Observation and clinical examination | Vascular |
| | Neurological |
| | Locomotor |
| | Skin and nails |
| | Footwear |
| Laboratory and hospital tests | Urinalysis |
| | Microbiology |
| | Blood tests |
| | History |
| | Gait analysis |
| | X-ray |
| | Other imaging techniques |
| | ECG |
| | Nerve conduction |

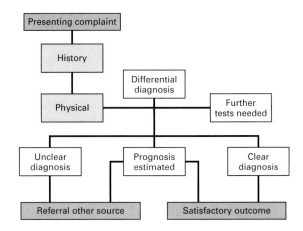

**Figure 1.1** The stages of assessment summarised.

possibilities. This approach focuses on symptom reduction and palliation.

A good assessment requires that the practitioner demonstrates good interviewing (communication) and observational skills. It is essential that the practitioner has effective listening skills and knows when and which questions to ask the patient (see Ch. 2). Research has shown that most diagnoses are based on observation and information volunteered by the patient (Sandler 1979).

Clinical, laboratory and hospital based tests provide additional data. Clinical tests involve physical examination of the patient (e.g. assessing ranges of motion at joints, taking a pulse) as well as near-patient tests such as assessing blood glucose levels with a glucometer. Most clinical tests are relatively quick and inexpensive to carry out and in most instances give fairly reliable and valid results. Technological advances mean that there are an increasing number of available clinical tests. Tests in laboratories and hospitals are more expensive and can be time-consuming. Such tests should only be used when it is necessary to confirm a suspected diagnosis, in cases of differential diagnosis or when the outcome of the test will have a positive influence on treatment.

### Risk assessment

Risk assessment can serve two purposes:

- identify patients who need immediate attention
- serve as a predictor for those 'at risk'.

On account of the demands on time it is often necessary for the practitioner to differentiate between those patients who need immediate attention and those who do not. Table 1.2 summarises the presenting problems which should be given high priority. In clinics where there are lengthy waiting lists patients may be screened initially to assess whether they have one or more problems which appear in Table 1.2 and are then given immediate treatment.

The term 'at risk' usually denotes those patients at risk of developing ulceration and infection. Identifying those at risk is a complex task. Currently, research into risk factors related to lower limb problems is sparse and thus it is difficult to produce risk assessment methods that are robust and valid. Considerable research has been undertaken into the risk assessment of pressure ulcers (Lothian 1987). In relation to the lower limb some work has been undertaken into developing methods of risk assessment to identify diabetics at risk of developing diabetic ulcers (Zahra 1998). Further work is needed in this

**Table 1.2** Presenting problems which should be given high priority

| Problem | Features |
| --- | --- |
| Pain | Constant, weightbearing and non-weightbearing<br>Affects patient's normal daily activities |
| Infection | Raised temperature (pyrexia)<br>Sign of acute inflammation<br>Signs of spreading cellulitis<br>Lymphangitis, lymphadenitis |
| Ulceration | Loss of skin<br>May or may not be painful<br>May expose underlying tissues |
| Acute swelling | Unrelieved pain<br>Very noticeable swelling<br>May have associated signs of inflammation |
| Abnormal skin changes | Distinct colour change<br>Discharge may be malodorous<br>Itching<br>Bleeding |

whole area before such measures can be used with confidence.

## Making a diagnosis

Arriving at a diagnosis is a complex activity. Studies of clinical reasoning show that practitioners use one or more of the following approaches (Higgs & Jones 2000):

- hypothetico-deductive reasoning
- pattern recognition
- interpretative model.

Hypothetico-deductive reasoning is based on generating hypotheses using clinical data and knowledge. These hypotheses are tested through further inquiry during the assessment. The evidence gained is evaluated in relation to existing knowledge and a conclusion reached on the basis of probability (Gale 1982).

Pattern recognition is a process of recognising the similarity between a set of signs and symptoms. The important aspect of the use of categorisation in clinical reasoning is the link practitioners make between the pattern they are currently observing and previous cases showing the same or similar patterns.

The interpretative model is very different from the other two models. This approach is based on the practitioner gaining a deep understanding of the patient's perspective and the influence of contextual factors. Protagonists of this approach believe that the meaning patients give to their problems, including their understanding of and their feelings about their problem, can significantly influence their levels of pain tolerance, disability and the eventual outcome (Ferurestein & Beattie 1995).

Studies have shown that with all these approaches there is an association between clinical reasoning and knowledge (Higgs & Jones 2000). There is a symbiotic relationship between the knowledge base of practitioners and their clinical reasoning ability. It is not possible to develop problem-solving skills in the absence of cognitive knowledge related to the specific problem.

There are three partners in the assessment process; the practitioner, the patient and the wider environment. The ability of a practitioner to undertake an effective assessment and make a diagnosis is influenced by a range of factors:

- personal values, beliefs and perceptions
- knowledge base related to the problem(s)
- reasoning skills (cognition and metacognition)
- previous clinical experience
- familiarity with similar cases.

There can be enormous differences between practitioners, both in their assessment findings and their diagnoses. For example, Comroe & Botelho (1947) described a study in which 22 doctors were asked to examine 20 patients and note whether cyanosis was present. Under controlled conditions these patient were assessed for cyanosis by oximeter. When the results of the clinical assessment were compared with the oximeter results, it was found that only 53% of the doctors diagnosed cyanosis in subjects with extremely low oxygen content: 26% said cyanosis was present in subjects with normal oxygen content. Curran & Jagger (1997) found poor agreement between podiatrists when diagnosing common conditions of the leg and foot. Agreement improved when a patient expert system was used. Expert patient systems are increasingly being used, in particular in medicine (Adams et al 1986). These computer-based systems provide practitioners with a wealth of information and are used to guide and direct clinical decision making.

Unfortunately, making a diagnosis is not a precise science: errors can and do occur. Practitioners should always keep an open mind when making a diagnosis, reflect on the process they have used, keep up to date with current literature and technology and request a second opinion when unsure.

Sometimes the practitioner may have generated more than one possible diagnosis; in these instances the practitioner has to undertake a differential diagnosis, i.e. decide which is the most likely from a number of possibilities. When arriving at a differential diagnosis the practitioner should take into account the factors listed in Table 1.3. For example, a number of conditions affect specific age groups (e.g. the osteochon-

**Table 1.3** Factors which should be taken into consideration when making a differential diagnosis

| Social history | Age |
| --- | --- |
| | Gender |
| | Race |
| | Social habits |
| | Occupation |
| | Leisure pursuits |
| Medical history | Family history |
| | Medication |
| Symptoms | Onset |
| | Type of pain |
| | Aggravated by/relieved by |
| | Seasonal variation |
| Signs | Site |
| | Appearance |
| | Symmetry |
| Specific tests | Imaging techniques |
| | Urinalysis |
| | Microbiology |
| | Blood analysis |
| | Biopsy |
| | Foot pressure analysis |
| | Electrical conductive studies |

droses), whereas other conditions have specific presenting features (e.g. the sudden, acute, nocturnal pain associated with gout).

The patient is the key partner in the assessment process. Some patients want to play a greater role in decision making and their health care management. Additionally, patients are increasingly being seen as consumers of health care. As such, they have expectations of the type and quality of the health services they receive.

Patients' perceptions, beliefs and expectations related to their lower limb problems can be influenced by the following factors:

- home environment
- work environment
- culture
- socioeconomic status
- language skills
- general state of health.

The above factors can affect patients' needs, communication skills and, ultimately, the choices they make.

The wider health environment and context cannot be ignored in the assessment process.

- Don't ask the patient more than one question at a time. For example, if asking a closed-type question do not say, 'Could you tell me when you first noticed the condition, when the pain is worse and what makes it better?'. By the end of the question the patient will have forgotten the first part.
- Attempt to get the patient to give you an honest answer using his or her own words. Avoid putting words into the patient's mouth.
- Clarify inconsistencies in what the patient tells you.
- Get the patient to explain what he means by using certain terms, e.g. 'nagging pain'. Your interpretation of this term may differ from the patient's.
- Pauses are an integral part of any communication. They allow time for participants to take in and analyse what has been communicated and provide time for a response to be formulated. Allow the patient time to think how he wishes to answer your question. Avoid appearing as if you are undertaking an interrogation.
- In the early stages of the interview it is often better to use the term 'concern' rather than 'problem'. Asking patients what concerns them may elicit a very different response from asking them what the problem is. Some patients may feel they do not have a problem as such but are worried about some symptom or sign they have noticed. Asking them what concerns them may get them to reveal this rather than a denial that they have any problems.
- Asking personal and intimate questions can be very difficult. Do not start the interview with this type of question; wait until further into the interview when hopefully the patient is more at ease with you. Try to avoid showing any embarrassment when asking an intimate question as this may well make the patient feel uncomfortable.
- It is important that the patient understands why you are asking certain questions. Remember that the assessment interview is a two-way process: besides gathering information from the patient it can be used for giving information to him.
- Some patients, on account of a range of circumstances such as deafness, speech deficit or language difference, may not be able to communicate with the practitioner. In these instances it is important that the practitioner involves someone known to the patient to communicate on his behalf, e.g. relative, friend or carer.
- The patient may have difficulty listening and interpreting what you are saying through fear, anxiety, physical discomfort or mental confusion. Be aware of non-verbal and verbal messages that can give clues to the patient's emotional state.

## Listening skills

Listening is an active not a passive skill. Many people ask questions but do not listen to the response. A common example is the general introductory question: 'How are you?'. Most responses tend to be in the affirmative: 'Fine', 'OK'. Occasionally, someone responds by saying they have not been too well, only to get the response from the supposed listener: 'Great; pleased to hear everything is fine'. Similarly, do not limit your attention to that which you want to hear or expect to hear. Listen to all that is being said and watch the patient's non-verbal behaviour. The average rate of speech is 100–200 words a minute; however, we can assimilate the spoken word at around 400 words per minute. As a result the listener has 'extra time' to understand and interpret what is being said. If you have asked a question you should listen to *all* of the answer. Often when trying to understand the clinical nature of a patient's problem, there is a great temptation to listen to the first part of an answer and then to immediately use this information to try and make a diagnosis. This may mean that you are not paying careful attention to important clinical information, which the patient may give, at the end of their reply. Finally, it is important that you don't let your mind wander on to unrelated thoughts such as what you are going to do after the interview. Before you know it you have missed a good chunk of what the patient has been telling you and have most probably missed important and relevant information.

In order to be a good listener you need to set aside your own personal problems and worries and give your full attention to the other person. It is inevitable that, at times, one's attention does wander. This may be due to lack of concentration, tiredness or because the patient has been allowed to wander off the point. In the case of the former do not be afraid to say to the patient, 'Sorry, could I ask you to go over that again?'. In the latter case, politely interrupt the patient and use your questioning skills to bring the conversation back to the subject in hand.

During the interview the techniques of paraphrasing, reflection and summarising can be used to aid listening and ensure you understand what the patient is trying to convey.

**Paraphrasing.** This technique is used to clarify what a person has just said to you in order to get him to confirm its accuracy or to encourage him to enlarge. It involves re-stating, using your own and the patient's words, what the patient has said.

**Reflection.** This technique is similar to prompting in that it is used to encourage the patient to continue talking about a particular issue that may involve feelings or concerns. It may be used when the patient appears to be reluctant to continue or is 'drying up'. It involves the practitioner repeating in the patient's own words what the patient has just said.

**Summarising.** This technique is used to identify what you consider to be the main points of what the patient is trying to tell you. It can also be a useful means of controlling the interview when a patient continues to talk at length about an issue. To summarise, the practitioner draws together the salient points from the whole conversation. At the end of the summary the patient may agree with, add to or make corrections to what the practitioner has said. Summarising serves a useful purpose in checking the validity, clarity and understanding of old information; it does not aim to develop new information.

The basic skills of a good listener are highlighted in Table 2.2.

**Table 2.2** Skills of a good listener

- Look at the patient when he/she starts to talk
- Use body language such as nodding, leaning forward to demonstrate to the speaker that you are interested in what is being said
- Do not keep looking at the time
- Adopt a relaxed posture
- Use paraphrasing, reflecting and summarising to show the patient that you are listening to and understanding what he/she is/are saying

## Non-verbal communication skills

This involves all forms of communication apart from the purely spoken (verbal) message. It is through this medium that we create first impressions of people and, similarly, people make initial judgements about us. Once made, first impressions are often difficult to change, yet research has shown they are not always reliable. Therefore, it is particularly important that we consider non-verbal communication here since it affects not only how we are perceived when we communicate but also how we make judgements about the patient.

Non-verbal behaviour includes behaviours such as posture, touch, personal space, physical appearance, facial expressions, gestures and paralanguage (i.e. the vocalisations associated with verbal messages, such as tone, pitch, volume, speed of speech). It is said that we primarily communicate non-verbally. Remember the old adage 'a picture says a thousand words'. Your body language and paralanguage will send an array of messages to your patient prior to you saying anything. Non-verbal communication serves many useful purposes. It can be used to:

- replace, support or complement speech
- regulate the flow of verbal communication
- provide feedback to the person who is transmitting the message, e.g. looking interested
- communicate attitudes and emotions (Argyle 1972, Hargie et al 1994).

The average person only speaks for a total of 10–11 minutes daily, with the average spoken sentence lasting only around 2.5 seconds (Birdwhistell 1970). Therefore, non-verbal communication is the main mode of conveying our emotional state in most types of human interactions. In fact, in a typical conversation only one-third of the social meaning will be conveyed verbally – a full two-thirds is communicated through non-verbal channels! (Birdwhistell 1970).

Due to the broad literature in this area the following section will focus on selected aspects of non-verbal behaviour and how they may influence the success of the assessment interview. For the interested reader, there is a wide range of books available which look at the topic of non-verbal communication, many specialising in the clinical interaction: see Davis (1994), Dickson et al (1997), Hargie (1997), or the winter 1995 edition of the *Journal of Nonverbal Behavior* for further information on this topic.

**Eye contact.** Eye-to-eye contact is frequently the first stage of interpersonal communication. It is the way we attract the other person's attention. Direct eye-to-eye contact creates trust between two people; hence, the innate distrust felt of someone who avoids eye contact. However, we do not keep constant eye-to-eye contact throughout a conversation. The receiver looks at the speaker for approximately 25–50% of the time, whereas the speaker looks at the other person for approximately half as long. So in other words, people tend to look more at the other person when they are listening compared with when they are speaking.

Too much eye contact is interpreted as staring and is seen as a hostile gesture. Too little is interpreted as a lack of interest, attention or trustworthiness. Interviewers cannot afford to look inattentive because the patient may interpret this as meaning that he has said enough and as a result may stop talking. Conversely, withdrawing eye contact may be used as a legitimate way of getting the patient to stop talking.

Health care practitioners should be aware of the frequency and duration of eye contact they have with their patients. The use of eye contact is important for assessing a range of patient needs and providing feedback and support, and its use during the interview should be based on the pro-fessional judgement of the practitioner (Davidhizar 1992). Certainly eye-to-eye contact is recommended at the beginning of the interview, to gain rapport and trust, and at the end of the interview by way of closing the interview. However, you should always be aware of potential cultural and gender differences in appropriate level of eye contact. For example, Hall (1984) has reported that on average women tend to make more eye-to-eye contact compared with men, so adjust your non-verbal behaviour accordingly.

**Facial expression.** Facial expression is arguably the most important form of human communication next to speech itself (Hargie et al 1994). It is via our facial expression we communicate most about our emotional state, and the meaning of a wide range of facial expressions (e.g. happy or sad) are recognised universally (Ekman & Fresen 1975). Smiling, together with judicious eye-to-eye contact, signifies a receptive and friendly persona and inspires a feeling of confidence and friendliness. Facial expressions often carry even more weight in a social interaction than the spoken word. For example, if a practitioner is giving a very positive verbal message to the patient but, at the same time, the practitioner's facial expression communicates anxiety and doubt, then it is likely that the patient will pay more attention to the facial message. This is because verbal behaviour is much easier to control than non-verbal and, as a result, non-verbal communication is likely to be more honest! Therefore, it is important that practitioners are always aware of the message they are communicating using their facial expressions.

**Posture and gestures.** The manner in which we hold ourselves and the way in which we move says a lot about us as individuals. This area of non-verbal behaviour is often referred to as *kinesics* and includes all those movements of the body which complement the spoken word (e.g. gestures, limb movements, head nods, etc.). One particularly important aspect is posture. Four types of posture have been identified:

- *approaching posture*, which conveys interest, curiosity and attention, e.g. sitting upright and slightly forward in a chair facing towards the person you are communicating with

- *withdrawal posture*, which conveys negation, refusal and disgust, e.g. distance between the receiver and the communicator, shuffling, gestures indicating agitation
- *expansion*, which conveys a sense of pride, conceit, mastery, self-esteem, e.g. expanded chest, hands behind head with shoulders in air, erect head and trunk
- *contraction*, which conveys depression, dejection, e.g. sitting in a chair with head drooped, arms and legs crossed or head held in hands, avoiding eye contact.

Clearly, the posture adopted by the health care practitioner is important in developing a rapport and a working therapeutic relationship with the patient.

When we speak we also tend to use our arms and hands to reinforce and complement the verbal message. In fact, when people are constrained from using their arms and hands, they experience greater difficulty in communicating (Riseborough 1981). Self-directed gestures such as ring twisting, self-stroking and nail biting may indicate anxiety. Be aware of self-participation in these types of activities as you may convey a non-verbal message of anxiety to your patient while verbally you are trying to convey a confident approach. The health care profession should be sensitive to the non-verbal gestures used by the patient as these may reveal more about the patient's thoughts and feelings than they are able to communicate verbally (Harrigan & Taing 1997).

**Touch.** The extent to which touching is permissible or encouraged is related to culture (McDaniel & Andersen 1998). In general, the British people are not known as a nation of 'touchers'. During the assessment it may be necessary to touch the patient in order to examine a part of his body. This type of touching, known as functional touching, is generally acceptable to most patients as part of the role of the practitioner and as such does not carry any connotation of a social relationship. However, people from certain cultures may find it difficult to accept, even in medical settings. Prior to functional touching of a patient, it is important that you inform the patient what you intend to do and the reasons for doing it.

During the interview you may wish to use touch as a means of reassuring the patient, to indicate warmth, show empathy or as a sign of care and concern (McCann & McKenna 1993). A hand lightly placed upon a shoulder or holding a patient's hand are means of showing concern and giving reassurance. It is difficult to produce guidelines for when this type of touching should or should not be used. Practitioners must feel confident and happy in its use, and must also take into account a multitude of communication cues from the patient before deciding whether it is or is *not* appropriate (Davidhizar & Newman 1997).

**Proxemics.** All of us have a sense of our own personal territory. When someone invades that territory, depending upon the situation, we can be fearful, disturbed or pleased and happy. As with touch, our sense of personal space is affected by culture. In some cultures individuals have a large personal space, whereas in others they have a very small personal space. Encroaching on someone else's personal space can be perceived as intimidation and, in the case of the assessment interview, may put patients on their guard. As a result the patient may become reluctant to disclose relevant information. Hall (1969) defined the four zones of personal space (Table 2.3).

**Table 2.3** Four zones of personal space (Hall 1969)

| Zone | Distance | Activities |
|---|---|---|
| Intimate | 0–0.5 metres | Intimate relationships/close friends |
| Personal | 0.5–1.2 metres | What is usually termed 'personal space' |
| Social/consultative | 1.2–3 metres | Distance of day-to-day interactions |
| Public | 3 metres + | Distance from significant public figures |

The zone in which people interact is highly influenced by social status and people who have an equal status tend to interact at closer distances (Zahn 1991). The assessment interview usually takes place in the social/consultative and the personal zone. During the interview it may be necessary to enter the intimate zone. Prior to doing this, notify the patient in order to justify any actions requiring closer contact.

Social interactions are not only influenced by distance, but also by bodily orientation. The angle at which you conduct the assessment interview may have a significant effect on the success of the interaction. There are four main ways in which you can position yourself in order to interact with the patient (Fig. 2.1): (i) conversation; (ii) cooperation; (iii) competition; and (iv) coaction. Research indicates that the conversation position is most appropriate for an assessment interview. In fact, research has shown that when GPs sat at a 90° angle to their patients during a clinical interview, the amount of

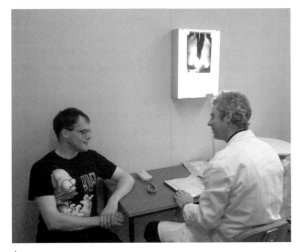

A

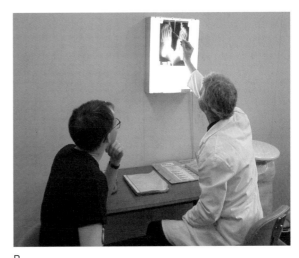

B

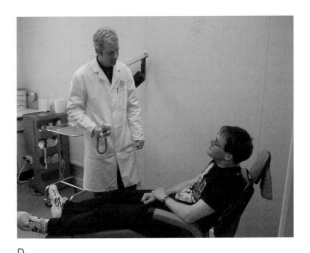

C

D

**Figure 2.1**  Body orientation may influence the success of the interview. The figures show four positions commonly encountered when two people interact. Which of the following orientations do you think would be most appropriate for the assessment interview?    **A.** Conversation    **B.** Cooperation    **C.** Competition    **D.** Coaction.

clinician–patient information exchanged increased by up to *six* times compared with when they interacted face-to-face (Pietroni 1976).

Clearly, the health care professional needs to be aware of the physical position they adopt when assessing a patient as this will have a significant impact on the kind of relationship they are hoping to achieve (Worchel 1986).

**Physical appearance.** We use our clothing and accessories to make statements about ourselves to others. Clothing can be seen as an expression of conformity or self-expression, comfort, economy or status. Uniforms are used as intentional means of communicating a message to others; often the message is to do with status. Uniforms are also used in the health care professions for cover and protection. Whether one wears a uniform (white coat, coloured top and trousers) for the assessment interview is open for debate, but one should pay attention to issues of cleanliness and appearance of dress, hair, hands, footwear and accessories such as jewellery – they all send messages to the patient. In addition to physical factors, which can be altered, you should also be aware of how 'non-changeable' physical characteristics may play a role in your interaction with the patient. For example, physically attractive and/or taller people are typically judged more favourably in general social interactions (Hensley & Cooper 1987, Melamed & Bozionelos 1992). Research has shown that within a health care environment, children make judgements about health care professionals on the basis of height. In general, taller health professionals were judged to be stronger and more dominant than their smaller colleagues, but they were not considered to be more intelligent nor more empathetic (Montepare 1995).

Finally, health care practitioners should also be aware of the impact of their appearance on any health promotion message that they hope to communicate. For example, the patient will often pay attention to the footwear worn by the practitioner. Avoid giving conflicting verbal and non-verbal messages, e.g. by wearing high-heeled slip-on shoes while advising patients that they should not wear this type of shoe.

**Paralanguage.** This involves the manner in which we speak. It includes everything from the speed at which we speak to the dialect we use. Paralanguage is the **bold**, underlining, *italics* and punctuation marks in our everyday speech! An individual who speaks fast is often considered by the receiver to be intelligent and quick, whereas a slow drawl may be associated with a lower level of intelligence. When talking to patients we should be careful not to speak too quickly as they will not understand what we say. Conversely, if speech is too slow, the patient may not have confidence in the practitioner.

When we speak we use pitch, intonation and volume to affect the message we transmit. Individuals who speak at a constant volume and do not use intonation and/or alter their pitch often come across as monotonous, dull and boring. Such speech is often difficult to listen to. Intonation and pitch should be used to highlight the important parts of your question and can be used to change the point you are trying to make. For example, in the following sentence you can see how changing the point of emphasis changes the message you are trying to get across.

- **You** must use the cream on your foot daily, i.e. *treatment is the responsibility of the patient.*
- You **must** use the cream on your foot daily, i.e. *it is essential that the treatment is carried out.*
- You must use the **cream** on your foot daily, i.e. *it is important that the cream is used and not some other substance.*
- You must use the cream on your **foot** daily, i.e. *the cream should be used on the foot and not some other part of the body.*
- You must use the cream on your foot **daily**, i.e. *treatment needs to be on a regular basis.*

The fluency with which we speak also tends to convey messages about mental and intellectual abilities. Repeated hesitations, repetitions, interjections of 'you know' or 'um' and false starts do not inspire confidence in the receiver (Christenfeld 1995). We all experience occasions when we are not as fluent as at other times. These occasions tend to occur when we are tired or under great stress. If possible, these times should be keep to a minimum during clinical assessment.

Dialect conveys which part of the country we originate from. It may also cause us to use vocabulary a person from another part of the country is not familiar with. Avoid using colloquial terms. Dialect, on the other hand, is not so easy to alter. The only time it should be considered is when patients cannot understand what the practitioner is saying. Finally, volume should not be changed too regularly. Shouting at the patient should be avoided. In the clinical setting, as in life in general, it certainly does not guarantee that the other person will listen more to what you say!

From this section it should be clear that health care professionals need to be sensitive to the kind of atmosphere they are creating through their non-verbal communication, and the role this may have in the subsequent interaction with the patient. The extent to which you establish a satisfactory rapport will depend heavily on your non-verbal skills and how you develop them in your clinical work (Grahe & Bernieri 1999).

## Stereotyping

Health care practitioners should be aware of their own underlying psychological characteristics, which may have a profound effect on the interaction – i.e. stereotypes. A stereotype is a belief that all members of a particular social group share certain traits or characteristics (Baron & Byrne 2000). For example, you might hold particular ideas about the characteristics of a patient who is an alcoholic, elderly, from an upper social class group, from a minority ethnic group or female. In fact, you probably already hold a range of stereotypes about a wide group of patients whom you have never actually treated! While stereotypes are not always negative, they do share a common characteristic in that they reduce the ability of the health care worker to see the patient as an *individual*. Consequently, any information gathered from the patient during the assessment interview is likely to be interpreted in the light of such stereotypes (Price 1987). Ganong et al (1987) conducted a review of 38 research studies, which examined stereotyping by nurses and nursing students. Results indicated that nurses held stereotypes about patients on the basis of age,

gender, diagnosis, social class, personality and family structure. However, the impact on actual patient care was harder to classify. What does seem to be the case is that patients were less likely to be seen as having unique concerns, health problems and social circumstances. Consequently, in addition to practising interviewing skills, it is important for health care practitioners to reflect on any belief systems they may hold regarding particular patient groups, and consider how such views may impair the overall success of the assessment interview.

## Documenting the assessment interview

It is essential either during or at the end of the assessment to make a permanent record of the findings of the interview. This record is essential as an aide-memoire for future reference when monitoring and evaluating the treatment plan and as a means of communicating your findings to another practitioner who may collaborate in treating the patient.

Despite recent discussions within the field of podiatry regarding changing to electronic data management systems, the majority of patient records are still stored on paper. However, the use of computerised records is on the increase, particularly in private practice. It may well be in the future that paper records are discarded completely, and replaced by computerised techniques. Whatever the future may hold, the need for clear, accurate recording of information will still be the same. The recording of assessment findings, together with the recording of treatment provided, forms a legal document. Patient records would certainly be used if action was taken by a patient against a practitioner, or if certain agencies required detailed evidence of management and progress in the case of disability awards.

Patient records may take a variety of forms: at the simplest level a plain piece of paper may be used. If using plain paper it is essential to adopt an order to the presentation of your assessment findings: e.g. name, address, doctor, age, sex, weight, height, main complaint, medical history, etc. This is considered further in Chapter 5. A variety of patient record cards exist in the NHS and private practice. Many practitioners and health authorities produce their own tailor-made record card. The Association of Chief Chiropody Officers produced a standard record in 1986 for charting foot conditions, diagnoses and treatment progress.

Handwritten recording of information requires the following:

- The writing is legible and in permanent ink, not pencil. If another practitioner cannot read your writing the information is of no use.
- The information is set in a clear and logical order. It is essential to use an accepted method.
- Accurate recording of location and size of lesions or deformities. The use of prepared outlines of the feet are very good for indicating anatomical sites and save additional writing.
- Abbreviations are avoided where possible. What is obvious to you may not be so obvious to another practitioner.
- Entries are dated. Recording the medication a patient is taking is useless unless it is dated. Once dated the information can be updated as and when there is a change.
- Each entry should be signed and dated by the practitioner.

## STRUCTURING THE ASSESSMENT INTERVIEW

### Preparation

In order to achieve a good assessment interview it is essential you prepare yourself for the interview. The following should be taken into consideration.

**Purpose.** It is essential that the practitioner is clear as to the purpose of interview. In some instances the assessment interview may be used as a screening mechanism to identify patients for further assessment. It may be used to gain information from patients in order that their needs can be prioritised and those judged to be urgent can be seen first. On the other hand, the assess-

ment interview may be aimed at undertaking a full assessment of the patient, with treatment provided at the end of the interview.

**Letter of application.** Was the patient referred or self-referred? If the patient was referred by another health care practitioner there should be an accompanying letter of referral. Read this carefully so you are fully informed of the reasons for referral. This information should be used as a starting point for the assessment. If patients have referred themselves directly (self-referred) they should complete any appropriate documentation prior to the interview. Information on application forms can be used to prioritise patients and ensure the most suitable practitioner sees them. If no application form or letter of referral is available the practitioner has very little information prior to the interview, possibly only the patient's name.

You may wish to give the patient a short health questionnaire to complete prior to the assessment (pp. 77–78). This questionnaire may be sent to the patient prior to the interview or the patient may be asked to fill it in on arrival. These questionnaires provide the practitioner with important information before the start of the interview. The patient should be allowed time to complete the questionnaire in order that he can think about his responses. The advantage of such a questionnaire is that the practitioner does not have to ask the patient a series of routine questions during the interview. However, some patients may be reluctant to fill in a form without having met the practitioner or reluctant to disclose information in writing.

Prior to the interview try to read all the information you have about the patient. You can then come across to the patient as well informed and as someone who has taken an interest in him.

**Patient expectations.** Does the patient know what to expect from the assessment interview? Some new patients, prior to attending their assessment appointment, are sent an information sheet or booklet explaining the purpose of the assessment interview and what will happen during it. Such an initiative is helpful. The cause of a poor interview may be that the patient's expectations of what will happen are very different from what actually happens. For example, a patient who expected immediate treatment and had not envisaged any need for history taking may well say, 'Why are you asking me all these questions?'. Table 2.4 highlights what should be contained in a patient information booklet.

**Waiting room.** Patients can spend a lot of time in the waiting room, especially if they arrive too early or are kept waiting due to unavoidable circumstances. Try sitting in the waiting room in your clinic. Look around you: how welcoming is it? The waiting room sets the scene for the rest of the interview. Where possible, ensure that it is in good decorative order, clean, with magazines to read and informative, eye-catching posters or pictures on the wall. Make the most of a captive audience to put over important health education information. TV monitors showing health promotion videos may be used.

The name of the practitioner displayed outside the clinic may be useful. Some clinics, like a number of high street banks, have a display of photographs with the names and titles of those within the department or centre.

**Interview room.** The assessment interview may be carried out in an office or in a clinic. Both have advantages and disadvantages. Using an office prevents the patient being put off by surrounding clinical equipment. It facilitates eye-to-eye contact by sitting in chairs, and provides a non-clinical environment. This is especially useful if

**Table 2.4** Information booklet for patients to read prior to the interview

---

The booklet should contain the following information:

- The purpose of the assessment interview
- How long the interview should take
- What will happen during the interview
- Specific information the patient may be asked to provide, e.g. list of current medication
- Specific items the patient may be asked to bring, e.g. footwear
- Examples of questions he/she is likely to be asked
- The possible outcomes of the assessment interview, e.g. whether the patient will receive treatment at the end of it.

The booklet may also contain a health questionnaire for the patient to complete and bring to the assessment interview.

---

treatment is not normally provided at the end of the assessment. On the other hand, using a clinic ensures that clinical equipment is readily to hand and the patient can be moved into different positions if there are controls on the couch.

During the interview you should ensure that you are not disturbed. If there is a phone in the room, redirect calls. Ensure the receptionist does not interrupt. While the patient is in the room you should be giving him your undivided attention. Constant disturbances not only makes the assessment interview a protracted occasion but also can prompt the patient into feeling that his problem is not worthy of your attention.

## The interview

When the patient enters the room, welcome him to the clinic, preferably by name. This personalises the occasion for the patient and at the same time ensures that you have the correct patient. If you have difficulty with the patient's name, ask politely how to pronounce it rather than doing so incorrectly. Introduce yourself. As part of the Patient's Charter you should be wearing a name badge but a personal introduction is usually preferable, especially if the patient's eyesight is poor. It is useful to shake the patient by the hand since touch is an important aspect of non-verbal behaviour (as discussed earlier), although this may be influenced by personal preference.

At this stage you may find it helpful to make one or two general conversation points about the weather, the time of year or some news item. This enables patients to see you as a fellow human. Remember that during the interview they are going to give a lot of themselves to you. It is important that patients feel you are someone they wish to disclose information to. Use the introduction as an opportunity to explain the purpose of the interview and what will happen.

The positioning of patient and practitioner can influence the success of the assessment interview. Ideally, you and the patient should be at the same level in order to facilitate eye-to-eye contact. Barriers such as desks are often used in medical interviews. They can be considered as means of making the interview formal. Standing over a patient who is sitting down or lying on a couch may be intimidating.

**Data gathering.** It is essential that the practitioner is clear as to what areas should be covered in the interview. A logical and ordered approach should be adopted. However, it is not always possible or desirable to stick to an ordered approach. Patients tend to talk around issues or elect to give information about a question that you asked earlier at the end of the interview. You must make allowances for this.

Effective and efficient use of time is paramount. Experienced practitioners combine the interview with the examination. This is achieved by, for example, feeling pulses and skin temperature while simultaneously asking questions about medical history. This technique is a matter of preference; some prefer to complete the interview before commencing the examination.

After each assessment interview reflect upon it. Ask yourself how you could improve your performance and how you could make better use of the time. This will help you to make the best use of the data-gathering stage of the interview. Peer appraisal is another mechanism that you may find helpful in aiding you to develop good data-gathering skills.

## Closure

Bringing the assessment interview to a close is a difficult task. When do you know you have enough information? This is a difficult question to answer. Some presenting problems, together with information from the patient, can be easily diagnosed. Other problems are not so easy to resolve and may require further questioning and investigations.

General medical practitioners have been shown to give their patients, on average, 6 minutes of their time. Psychotherapists, on the other hand, spend 1 hour or more on each assessment. Unfortunately the demands on practitioners' time means they are often not in a position to give the patient as much time as they would like.

As a general rule of thumb the interview should be brought to a close when the practitioner feels the patient has been given an opportunity to talk about the problem. Body language can be used to convey the closing of the interview. Standing up from a sitting position, shuffling of papers, withdrawing eye-to-eye contact are all ways by which the end of the interview can be conveyed to the patient, together with a verbal message.

The patient should not leave the interview without fully understanding what is to happen next and without an opportunity to ask questions. A range of outcomes may result from the assessment interview (Table 2.5). Patients should know which outcome applies to them. They should always be given the opportunity to raise any queries or concerns they may have prior to leaving the assessment. This is one of the most important parts of the assessment and should not be hurried. The patient must leave the assessment fully understanding the findings of the assessment interview and what action, if any, is to be taken, and it is the responsibility of the health care professional to ensure that they have communicated such information clearly (Calkins et al 1997).

It is helpful to provide written instructions as a follow-up to the interview. For example, if the patient is to be offered a course of treatment what will the treatment involve, when will it be given, who will give it, what problems may the patient experience?

**Table 2.5** Outcomes from the assessment interview

- Treatment is not required; the patient requires advice and reassurance
- The patient can look after the problem once appropriate self-help advice has been given
- A course of treatment is required; the patient should be informed as to whether treatment will commence straight after the assessment interview or at a later date
- The patient needs to be referred to another practitioner for treatment
- Further examination and investigations are required before a definitive diagnosis can be made
- A second opinion is required
- The urgency for treatment should be prioritised

## Confidentiality

The information the patient divulges during the interview is confidential. It should not be disclosed to other people unless the patient has given consent. The Data Protection Act 1998 requires that all personal data held on computers should be 'secure from loss or unauthorised disclosure'. The General Medical Council (1991) and the National Health Service (1990) have laid down guidelines on confidentiality.

## WHAT MAKES A GOOD ASSESSMENT INTERVIEW?

The prime purpose of the assessment interview is to draw out information, experiences and opinions from the patient. It is the duty of the interviewer to guide and keep the interview to the subject in hand. At the same time, it is equally important to encourage the patient to talk and to clear up any misunderstandings as you go along. Keeping the balance between these two competing aims is not an easy task. One way of checking on this is to ask yourself who is doing most of the talking. Is it you or the patient? If you are to achieve the aims of the assessment interview it should be the patient.

It is not essential that you like the patient you are interviewing. What is important is that you adopt a professional approach, demonstrate empathy and deal with the patient in a competent and courteous manner. It is essential that you do not make value judgements based on your own biases and prejudices. Respect the patient; avoid stereotyping. Do not jump to conclusions before reaching the end of the interview.

As highlighted earlier, the assessment interview should be patient-centred; its prime purpose is to gain information from the patient. However, one sometimes comes across patients who appear unable to stop talking. What can the practitioner do in these instances?

The first question to ask is why the patient is talking so much. Is it because he is lonely and welcomes the opportunity to talk, is he very self-centred, is he avoiding telling you what the real concern is by talking about minor issues? The reason will influence the action you take. If you feel the patient wants to tell you something but is finding it difficult, try reflecting or summarise what you think has been said. Ask if there is anything else the patient would like to discuss. Encourage patients by telling them that you want to be able to help as much as you can; the more they tell you about their concerns the more you can help them.

On the other hand, if you feel you need to control a talkative patient you may find the following techniques helpful:

- use eye contact and your body language to inform the patient that you are bringing a particular section of the interview to a close
- politely interrupt the patient, summarise what he has said and say what is to happen next
- ask questions that bring the patient back to the topic under discussion.

The converse of talkative patients are those who are reluctant to disclose information about themselves. This may be because they do not see the purpose of the questions you are asking, they are shy, they cannot articulate their concerns, they are fearful of what the outcomes may be or they are too embarrassed to disclose certain information. Your response will depend on the cause of the reticence.

Explaining why you need to know certain information will be helpful if the patient is hesitant. For example, a patient may wonder why you need to know what medication he is taking when all he wants is to have a corn treated. If you feel the patient cannot articulate what he wants to say, you may find that closed questions can help. This type of questioning limits responses but can be helpful for a patient who has difficulty putting concerns and problems into words. You need to use a range of closed questions and avoid leading questions if you are to ensure you reach an accurate diagnosis.

The shy or embarrassed person may find self-disclosure very difficult. It has been shown that people tend to disclose more about themselves as they get older. In general, females disclose more than males. When privacy is ensured and the interviewer shows empathy, friendliness and acceptance, patients have been shown to disclose more information. Reciprocal disclosure can also be helpful.

**Feedback.** In order to develop your interview technique it is important that you obtain feedback on your performance. Mention has already been made of self- and peer assessment of the interview. This is a valuable process, which should be ongoing. Patient feedback is another valuable mechanism. Questionnaires (postal or self-administered) and structured or unstructured interviews are ways in which patient reactions to the interview can be obtained. Suggestions as to how to improve interviews should be welcomed.

## SUMMARY

The interview is the process of initiating an assessment of the lower limb. The relationship created between the practitioner and the patient during the interview will hopefully lead to an effective diagnosis. A good interview can provide the majority of the information required without having to resort to numerous tests and unnecessary examination. There is no one formula that can be applied to all assessment interviews. Each patient should be treated as an individual with specific needs. Practitioners should develop their interviewing skills in order that the interview achieves a successful outcome for the patient and the practitioner.

## REFERENCES

Argyle M 1972 The psychology of interpersonal behaviour. Penguin, Harmondsworth

Authier J 1986 Showing warmth and empathy. In: Hargie O (ed) A handbook of communication skills. Routledge, London

Baron R A, Byrne D 2000 Social psychology, 9th edn. Allyn & Bacon, Boston

Birdwhistell R L 1970 Kinesics and context. University of Pennsylvania Press, Philadelphia

Byrne P, Long E 1976 Doctors talking to patients: A study of verbal behaviour of general practitioners consulting in their surgeries. HMSO, London

Calkins D, Davis R, Reiley P et al 1997 Patient–physician communication at hospital discharge and patients' understanding of the postdischarge treatment plan. Archives of Internal Medicine 157: 1026

Christenfeld N 1995 Does it hurt to say Um. Journal of Nonverbal Behavior 19: 171

Data Protection Act 1998 EC Data Protection Directive (95/46 EC)

Davidhizar R 1992 Interpersonal communication: a review of eye contact. Infection Control and Hospital Epidemiology 13: 222

Davidhizar R, Newman J 1997 When touch is not the best approach. Journal of Clinical Nursing 6: 203

Davis C 1994 Patient practitioner interaction: An experiential manual for developing the art of healthcare, 2nd edn. Slack Inc, New Jersey

Dickson D, Hargie O, Morrow N 1997 Communication skills training for health professionals, 2nd edn. Chapman & Hall, London

Ekman P, Fresen W V 1975 Unmasking the face. Prentice-Hall, Englewood Cliffs, New Jersey

Ganong L H, Bzdek V, Manderino M A 1987 Stereotyping by nurses and nursing students: a critical review of research. Research in Nursing and Health 10: 49

General Medical Council 1991 Professional conduct and discipline: Fitness to practice. GMC, London

Grahe J, Bernieri F 1999 The importance of nonverbal cues in judging rapport. Journal of Nonverbal Behavior 23: 253

Hall E T 1969 The hidden dimension. Doubleday, New York

Hall J A 1984 Nonverbal sex differences: communication accuracy and expressive style. Johns Hopkins University, Baltimore

Hargie O 1997 The handbook of communication skills, 2nd edn. Routledge, London

Hargie O, Saunders C, Dickson D 1994 Social skills in interpersonal communication, 3rd edn. Routledge, London

Hargie O, Dickson D, Boohan M, Hughes K 1998 A survey of communication skills training in UK schools of medicine: present practices and prospective proposals. Medical Education 32: 25

Harrigan J, Taing K 1997 Fooled by a smile: detecting anxiety in others. Journal of Nonverbal Behavior 21: 203

Hensley W, Cooper R 1987 Height and occupational success: a review and critique. Psychological Reports 60: 843

McCann K, McKenna H P 1993 An examination of touch between nurses and elderly patients in a continuing care setting in Northern Ireland. Journal of Advanced Nursing 18: 38

McDaniel E, Andersen P 1998 International patterns of interpersonal tactile communication. Journal of Nonverbal Behavior 22: 59

Melamed J, Bozionelos N 1992 Managerial promotion and height. Psychological Reports 71: 587

Montepare J 1995 The impact of variations in height in young children's impressions of men and women. Journal of Nonverbal Behavior 19: 31

National Health Service Circular No 1990 (Gen) 22, 7 June 1990 A code of practice on the confidentiality of personal health information. London

patient's own words what she is concerned about and what she sees as a problem. Avoid medical jargon wherever possible.

Having obtained an idea of the patient's concerns, it may help to find out if she has any thoughts as to the cause. Ask the reason for such conclusions. The answers to these questions may reveal whether patient and practitioner share the same view.

When patients do reveal what is worrying them, avoid being judgemental and making comments such as 'Oh, that's nothing!' or 'I don't know why you are so worried!'. Remember it is a problem to the patient even if it is relatively innocuous to you. Patients may not reveal their real reason for coming to see you until they are just about to leave. This can be a source of annoyance to the busy practitioner. Do try and give the patient time even if it is at the end of the consultation.

## Patients with special needs

Some patients may experience other difficulties in telling you about their concerns and problems than simply having poor powers of description. The patient may be deaf and dumb, have suffered a stroke, have a speech impediment or have learning or language difficulties. It is important you give these patients extra time. Avoid jumping to too many assumptions. If the patient can write, ask her to write down the nature of the complaint. Friends or relatives may be able to provide valuable details and information or act as interpreters.

## Why did the patient seek your help?

A variety of factors can influence why a patient has chosen to visit your practice. Table 3.2 gives the usual reasons for a patient choosing a particular practitioner. It is important to find out what made the patient choose you. For example, a patient who has been referred by a friend or relative may find it very easy to disclose her concerns to you. The friend/relative may have been very complimentary about your abilities. On the other hand, a patient who is seeking a second opinion

**Table 3.2**  Reasons for a patient choosing a practitioner

- Applied for treatment at their local health service
- Found your name in the yellow pages
- Saw an advertisement
- Noticed your plate outside the practice
- Were advised by a friend or relative to seek your help
- Were referred by another health practitioner, e.g. GP
- Are seeking a second opinion because they were unhappy with the response of the first practitioner

may want you to give a different diagnosis from the one given by the previous practitioner. As a result she may not disclose all the salient features of the problem. It is important to remember that outstanding legal claims for lower limb injuries may affect the patient's perspective.

## ASSESSMENT OF THE PROBLEM

Assessment of the problem involves acquiring information about the history of the problem. The history must be taken logically and systematically. An assessment of the current level of pain and discomfort should also be undertaken.

## History of the problem

History taking involves finding answers to a range of questions (Table 3.3). Many diseases can be identified by the pattern of symptoms they display. Research has shown that history taking

**Table 3.3**  The history of the problem: questions to ask the patient

- Where is the problem?
- How did it start?
- How long have you had the problem?
- Where is the problem?
- When does it trouble you?
- What makes it worse?
- What makes it better?
- What treatments have you tried?
- Are you treating it at the moment?

can be more effective in diagnosing a problem than clinical tests alone (Sandler 1979).

**Where is the problem?** Locating the problem is very important. Getting the patient to show you by pointing is the best way. If the patient has difficulty reaching the area, you may find it helpful to present an outline of the lower limb and ask her to mark the area affected. For example, pain may start in one area but then radiate to other areas. Some problems may have a precise location; others may be far more diffuse or have multiple sites. These variations may yield helpful clues to diagnosis. Isolating a localised area in the case of pain can be very helpful in differentiating enthesopathy from the more general discomfort associated with congestion of the heel pad. During the physical examination you may touch the area and attempt to elicit the symptoms in order to make sure you have isolated the area. Do not forget to tell the patient that this is what you are going to do. Palpation should use no more pressure than necessary to elicit symptoms and isolate the particular anatomy affected. It is essential that you record, either on a diagram or in words, the location of the problem and give an indication in the records as to whether it is well localised or diffuse. For example, a patient with plantar digital neuritis (Morton's neuroma) may complain of acute pain at one particular site, but may also describe a paraesthesia which radiates towards the apex of the toes. Diagrams may be preferable to written descriptions. Another practitioner treating the patient on a different occasion can see exactly where the problem lies. It is essential that dimensions of skin lesions are recorded. This approach allows progress to be monitored for improvement or deterioration.

**How did it start?** It is important to identify how the problem started. The problem may have had a sudden or an insidious onset. For example, rheumatoid arthritis may have an acute sudden onset accompanied by raised temperature and severe joint pains, or more commonly a slow insidious onset with general aches and pains, which gradually get worse and more regular. Besides trying to locate the start of the condition, it is also important to record the symptoms the patient initially experienced. For example, was there anything visible at the start, such as a rash, swelling or erythema? Were there any symptoms, e.g. the throbbing associated with acute inflammation? Initial symptoms may be different from the patient's current symptoms, especially if the condition had an acute onset but is now chronic.

**How long have you had the problem?** It may be necessary to jog the patient's memory, especially if the problem started some time ago. Using family occasions such as weddings or births, national events or the season of the year may help the patient to pinpoint which time of the year it started.

**When does it trouble you?** Some conditions may give rise to constant symptoms. Others may occur especially at night or during the day. For example, one of the distinguishing features of gout is nocturnal pain. Chronic ischaemia is associated with pain in the calf muscle (intermittent claudication) after a period of walking and the maximum distance the patient can walk prior to experiencing pain gives an indication of the severity of the problem.

**What makes it worse and what makes it better?** Some conditions may improve on rest, others can deteriorate. Patients may discover all sorts of ways to alleviate their symptoms, e.g. wearing particular shoes, adopting a different walking pattern. Such information can provide valuable clues. In instances where patients alter their gait because of a problem affecting one part of their foot or leg they may develop secondary problems elsewhere. It is essential that the practitioner identifies the original problem, as treatment for the secondary problem will not be successful until the initial problem is identified.

**What treatments have you tried? Are you treating it at the moment?** It is important to find out if the patient has or is presently using any medications. Sometimes treatments can mask or alter the clinical features of a problem and make diagnosis difficult. For example, using 1% hydrocortisone cream on a fungal infection of the skin may mask the inflammatory response and blur the distinctive border between infected and non-infected areas.

It is important that you record the information the patient gives you in response to all these questions. All critical events should be dated.

## Dimensions of pain

Pain is a subjective, multidimensional phenomenon that can be affected by social and psychological factors. In the same way as individuals differ over what they perceive as a problem, individuals also differ when it comes to the assessment of their pain. Pain caused by apparently similar conditions affects individuals in very different ways. Practitioners should avoid making assumptions about the severity of pain an individual is experiencing. Patients vary in their abilities to cope with pain. Some are more than willing to complain about mild discomfort, whereas others make no complaint despite being in considerable pain.

Tolerance and coping are subjective concepts that are difficult to quantify. A patient's state of mind and personal circumstances may make their pain worse or demand that they ignore it. For example, it is well known that runners may continue to run in a race despite having sustained an injury.

The assessment of pain requires information about its character, distribution, severity, duration, frequency and periodicity. This information, coupled with the history of the problem and details of the patient's concerns, helps the practitioner to arrive at the correct diagnosis and draw up an effective treatment plan.

### Character

Pain can be superficial or deep. Pain arising in the skin often gives rise to a pricking sensation if brief or burning if protracted. Deep pain is more nebulous and is often associated with a dull ache. Patients may use a variety of adjectives to describe their pain (Table 3.4).

### Distribution

Pain may be localised, diffuse or radiating. Initially, a problem may give rise to localised pain but as it becomes chronic and the disease process spreads it can affect a wider area. Radiating pain can result from the extent of the disease or from pain being referred from one site to another; for example, a trapped spinal nerve can lead to pains in the leg. Usually, referred pain does not get worse when direct pressure is applied to the site affected. However, if the pain has a localised cause it usually worsens when direct pressure is applied.

### Severity

Certain conditions give rise to severe pain, e.g. myocardial infarction. However, a patient's ability to tolerate and cope with pain differs so much that a description of the severity of the pain must be assessed alongside the other features.

### Duration

Pain may be fleeting or may be persistent. Ascertaining the duration of the pain can provide valuable information. For example, pain due to intermittent claudication may last a few minutes to half an hour. The pain associated with a deep vein thrombosis is persistent. These differences can be helpful in differential diagnosis.

### Frequency and periodicity

Some conditions lead to pain occurring in a regular pattern; others result in a less predictable pain pattern. It may be that the pain recurs infrequently or regularly.

**Table 3.4** Descriptors used to describe pain

| | |
| --- | --- |
| Vice-like | Deep |
| Tooth ache | On touching |
| Throbbing | On weightbearing |
| Sharp | Intermittent |
| Stabbing | |
| Shooting | |
| Bursting | |

## Techniques for assessing pain

There are many general pain measures but there are no foot-specific pain measures that are widely used. Various foot-specific measures have been developed, but these have not resulted in general use. For example, Budiman-Mak et al (1991) developed the Budiman-Mak Foot Function Index. This index was used in elderly patients with rheumatoid arthritis to assess activity limitation, perceived difficulty and pain.

Weir et al (1998) in a survey of podiatrists found that 53% of podiatrists did not assess their patient's foot pain. This is of concern, as the accurate assessment of pain is critical for the identification of suitable and effective interventions.

A range of techniques can be used to provide more objective information about the dimensions of pain experienced by a patient.

**Numerical pain rating scales.** Different dimensions such as severity, frequency and duration can be assessed. For example, a patient may be asked to score the frequency of her pain using a 1–5 scale, where 1 signifies persistent, present all the time, and 5 is very infrequent, less than twice a week.

**Verbal descriptor scales (VDS).** Descriptive scales can also be used. The following descriptors can assess severity: slight, quite a lot, very bad, agonising. Verbal descriptor scales are reliant on the ability of patients to use words that best describe their pain. It is not possible to compare the descriptors used by individual patients.

**Visual analogue scales (VAS).** These scales can be used to assess the severity of pain. The technique involves asking the patient to indicate how severe their problem is. Figure 3.1 illustrates two different types of visual analogue scale.

The VAS records the intensity of pain and is more useful for acute rather than chronic pain. The VAS has many advantages (Weir et al 1998):

- subjective measure of pain intensity
- clear to the patient what is being measured
- has face validity as it appears relevant to the patient
- quick and easy to administer
- requires minimal training of the patient
- can be used in a variety of clinical settings including home visits
- high degree of reliability when used on the same patient
- useful indicator to compare 'before and after' situations (Bowsher 1994).

The VAS is not suitable for those with poor visual and motor coordination. It is thought to be unsuitable for elderly patients, as they may be confused and unable to adapt to the abstract thinking required (Hayes 1995). Rather than using a horizontal line a vertical line has been used, which is more akin to a thermometer (painometer). It has been argued that this approach facilitates the conceptualisation of pain increasing and may be easier to respond to than the horizontal scale (Herr & Mobily 1991).

**General pain questionnaires.** The most well-known general pain questionnaire is the McGill Pain Questionnaire, which is based on a 78-item structured questionnaire that provides information about present pain intensity and pain rating index. Use of this questionnaire indicates that a patient who describes their pain as frightening usually does not understand what is causing it (Melzack 1975). The use of this questionnaire has been criticised for the time it takes to complete and evaluate.

**Body-part questionnaires.** These questionnaires usually relate to pain in a particular anatomical part, e.g. Boeckstyns (1987) developed a knee pain questionnaire.

**Charts.** Charts can be used for patients to indicate where the pain occurs and, by using

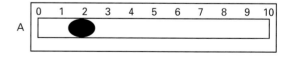

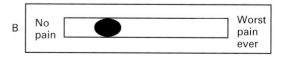

**Figure 3.1** Visual analogue scales **A.** Numerical **B.** Descriptive.

cators of the status of an ulcer and whether it is improving or deteriorating.

# Semi-quantitative measurement

Semi-quantitative measurement techniques usually involve an association of quantitative and qualitative methods. They are extremely varied in their design and application and represent attempts to quantify clinical observations where real quantitative methods are not appropriate, or as a cost-effective alternative. This type of measurement allows a common objective approach to obtaining, recording and communicating information. Results based on objective measurements tend to be modified and supported as more data are acquired (Calnan 1989). The following techniques exemplify some principles of semi-quantitative measurement.

## Rating (grading) scales

Scores are allocated to each of a logical order of observations, with each score in some way being better or worse than another. The scale may indicate, for instance, the level of function of some system or activity, and range from normal function to absence of function. The Medical Research Council (MRC) grading for muscle strength (Table 4.1) allocates scores from 0 to 5 to classify function in patients with peripheral nerve damage. This is considered in Chapter 8 as part of essential orthopaedic assessment.

The six ratings or gradings are placed in rank order of increasing muscle power, from 0 (no movement) to 5 (normal power). It is possible to record muscle power on a single occasion or, by taking a series of measurements, monitor improvement or deterioration in muscle power over time.

This type of data is classed as ordinal data. It is important to remember that the different scores on an ordinal scale cannot be compared in an arithmetic way because the intervals between the points on the scale are not equal. With reference to Table 4.1 it will be noted that the difference between 1 and 2 is not the same as the difference between 4 and 5. Also, a score of 4 is better than, but not twice as good as, a score of 2.

## Indices

Ankle–brachial, footprint and pulsility indices are commonly referred to in the literature. Each index is a ratio calculated from two quantitative values. The ankle–brachial index, for instance, is calculated by dividing the systolic ankle blood pressure by the systolic brachial pressure of the arm, e.g. $110/120 = 0.92$. Indices are often referred to as quantitative measures. Arguably they may best be considered as semi-quantitative measures because they lack two important characteristics of quantitative measures: indices are dimensionless, as they have no units of measurement, and their numerical values cannot be treated arithmetically. For example, comparison of indices should be treated in a similar way to ordinal data. An ankle–brachial index of 0.4 indicates a severe ischaemic condition but it cannot be said that the condition is twice as bad as an index of 0.8.

## Nominal categorisation

Nominal categorisation is essentially a very simple classification system where an observation is placed into one of two or more categories. The observation of interest could be either present or absent, and given arbitrary labels, perhaps A (present) and B (absent). For instance, a group of patients could be classified as hallux valgus present and hallux valgus absent. Data treated in this manner are described as nominal. This is the most basic level of data and gives the least amount of detail about an observation. The

**Table 4.1** Medical Research Council rating scale for muscle strength

| Rating | Characteristic |
| --- | --- |
| 0 | No movement |
| 1 | Palpable contraction but no visible movement |
| 2 | Movement but only with gravity eliminated |
| 3 | Movement against gravity |
| 4 | Movement against resistance, but weaker than the other side |
| 5 | Normal power |

hallux valgus condition is denoted simply as present or absent with no indication as to the severity of the condition. Only the simplest of arithmetic calculations can be carried out, and the data can only be used in the weakest types of statistical test.

## Integration of the three types of measurement

In practice, techniques selected from the three types of measurement may be used together to obtain a comprehensive clinical picture. This is illustrated in Table 4.2 by discussion of the results of measurements obtained for a patient presenting with walking difficulties. The relevant case history concerns a fall 1 year previously when a fractured pelvis was sustained. Following healing and discharge from hospital, the left leg and foot have become progressively weaker.

**Qualitative measurement.** There appears to be a motor deficit in the anterior compartment of the leg. This may be due to impingement of a peripheral nerve related to the pelvic fracture. The lack of ankle dorsiflexion during the swing phase is being compensated proximally, by elevation of the trunk and excessive flexion of the hip and knee, so that the toes can clear the ground.

**Semi-quantitative measurement.** A score of 3 on the MRC muscle strength grading scale. This indicates the level of impairment of the anterior muscle group. There is a deficit of motor power. The patient can dorsiflex the foot against gravity but not against resistance of the practitioner's hand.

**Quantitative measurement.** Active dorsiflexion can be quantified with a goniometer, e.g. $-10°$ dorsiflexion. The measurement of $-10°$ dorsiflexion indicates that with maximum contraction of the anterior muscle group the foot still remains $10°$ plantarflexed at the ankle. With assistance from the practitioner the maximum range of dorsiflexion can be obtained ($-5°$). Although an additional $5°$ of dorsiflexion was obtained with the practitioner's help the foot remained plantarflexed at the ankle. Comparison with the unaffected ankle and known normal values will enable the practitioner to determine the extent of the reduction in ankle dorsiflexion and identify the probable cause. The calf may have shortened if there is a loss of power in the anterior antagonist muscle group. Future measurements can be used to quantify improvement or deterioration of ankle dorsiflexion.

The example above demonstrates the value of integrating quantitative, semi-quantitative and qualitative types of measurement. A complete picture of the case can be constructed where evidence from one type of measurement complements another. Evaluation of the evidence then enables the practitioner to infer the cause of the changes in gait pattern with more than a reasonable degree of confidence. A thorough understanding of the problem gained in this manner enables an appropriate diagnosis and management plan to be decided.

It could be argued that all measurements for the patient could have been quantitative. Gait analysis could have been recorded with video and the movements of the limb segments digitised to allow quantification. Muscle power could have been quantified with a dynamometer. Nevertheless, the example represents the most usual clinical situation where the practitioner

**Table 4.2** Assessment results

| Type of measurement | Method | Results |
| --- | --- | --- |
| Qualitative | Visual observation of gait | Stance phase: The left foot slaps noisily against the ground at each step Swing phase: The left foot is plantarflexed, the hip and knee are flexed excessively and there is upper body sway to the right |
| Semi-quantitative | MRC muscle strength grading scale | The anterior muscle compartment score of 3 (i.e. movement against gravity) |
| Quantitative | Goniometric measurement | Active ankle dorsiflexion $-10°$ Passive ankle dorsiflexion $-5°$ |

The type of pressure transducer used by each system should also be considered. Resistive, piezoelectric and capacitance sensors convert mechanical signals into electrical signals for processing. The characteristics of transducers must be matched to the type of data the practitioner wishes to collect. The principles of hysteresis and repeatability have already been described. Spacial resolution, sampling frequency and dynamic response are other important characteristics described below. Practitioners requiring further information are directed to a very comprehensive review of pressure sensors by Urry (1999).

**Spacial resolution.** This refers to the number of sensors in one square centimetre in a homologous matrix. If spacial resolution is low, smaller anatomical features such as the lesser metatarsal heads or toes may be missed because there is greater spacing between individual sensors. Some in-shoe methods do not have a matrix of sensors but a number of separate or discrete transducers giving a very low spacial resolution. Problems with accurate placement of these transducers on the skin overlying the metatarsal heads was highlighted by comparison with data from the F-Scan high-resolution matrix insole sensor (Lord et al 1992). The discrete transducers were shown to be out of position by as much as 20 mm.

**Sampling frequency.** This refers to the number of times each individual sensor is scanned during data collection. Events which occur very quickly in the stance phase of gait may be missed if sampling frequency is low. For walking a sampling frequency of 50 Hz (50 times per second) is appropriate, whereas a higher sampling rate of 200 Hz is required for running.

**The dynamic range.** This should permit sampling of both high and low pressures expected in the patient cohort. If this were not the case then pressures occurring outside the range would be missed. Particular care is required with neuropathic patients as very high pressures are likely to saturate the sensors at their upper limit. Conversely, the soling materials in trainer footwear may be very shock absorbent and very low pressures may be missed.

Measurement instrumentation is prone to ageing and wear and tear, increasing the potential for error. Obvious changes in mechanical instruments may be noticed where the measurement scale becomes difficult to read, or its components become damaged or loose. Electronic components tend to age less noticeably. Noise is generated by electrical circuitry and it tends to increase as equipment ages. Everyday examples of noise include the background hum of audio speakers, or interference with visual information on a display monitor, rather like the lines produced on a television screen as an unsuppressed motor vehicle passes by. It is important to ensure that intrinsic noise produced by the instrumentation and electrical equipment in the vicinity does not interfere significantly with measurements. Careful use, monitoring and maintenance of equipment is essential if clinically useful measurements are to be obtained.

## The practitioner

Errors made by the practitioner can be reduced if a good practitioner–patient relationship is established. Effective communication and patient compliance is essential. Efficiency and confidence are usually transferred to the patient through verbal and non-verbal communication channels. Instructions given to patients must be clear, so that they understand exactly what they must do. Children, ethnic minorities and the physically and mentally disabled usually require more careful and considered approaches. Adequate time must be allowed for the measurements to be completed satisfactorily.

### Qualitative measurements

Qualitative measurements involve an internal appreciation and processing of the observations made. Qualitative techniques are subjective in nature and mainly involve the perceptions of sight, hearing and touch. Some senses are more acute in some individuals than in others. Different life experiences, age, education, state of health or mind and environmental factors will affect these perceptions. Qualitative measurements are therefore more prone to bias errors in practitioners than are quantitative measures. An awareness of the problems associated with subjectivity is important, because different individuals may perceive the same observation in different ways.

Often, preconceived ideas lead to mistakes, as illustrated in Figure 4.2A. When first seen most people read the legends incorrectly as 'Paris in the spring', 'Once in a lifetime', and 'Bird in the hand'. We have a tendency to see what we expect to see and ignore what we consider unimportant. This may happen in diagnosis, when a feature associated with a particular condition is given greater importance than it should receive and assumptions lead to a rapid, poorly considered diagnosis. It may be that other clinical features indicate a different pathology but these may go unnoticed, be ignored or be regarded as of little significance. By remaining as objective as possible and adopting a systematic problem-solving approach this tendency will be reduced.

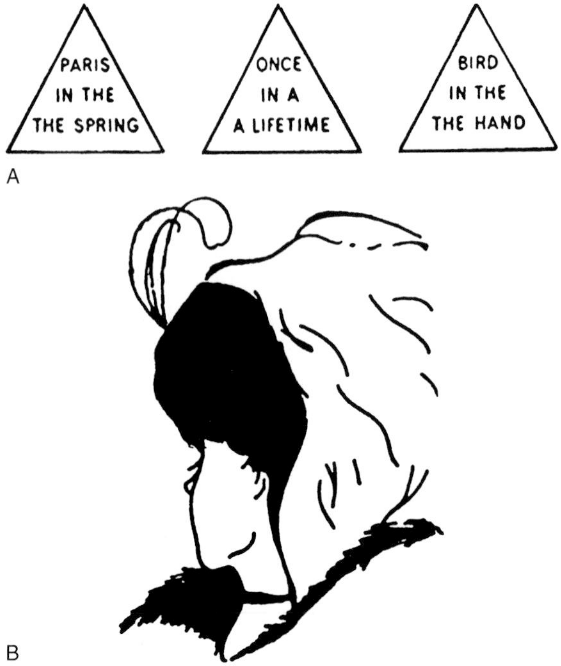

The brain may interpret the same observation in different ways, as shown in Figure 4.2B. The same observation may not only differ between individuals but differ in the same individual on different occasions or as they make a closer study.

Some quantitative measurement procedures depend on some subjective decisions by the practitioner. The location of pulses, anatomical landmarks and alignment of instrumentation all rely on subjectivity, thus increasing the potential for bias error. It is important to be aware of the subjective qualitative factors which may impair objective measurement so that attempts can be made to control them.

A

B

**Figure 4.2   A.** The three triangles. Failure to see the duplicated words is common. We see only what we want to see   **B.** How old is she? Some observers see a young woman, others an old woman. The chin and neck of the former become the nose and mouth of the latter and vice versa (Munro & Edwards 1990).

### Vision

Vision plays a major part in measurement. During clinical training a student practitioner develops a 'trained eye'. Recognition of pathology develops with time and practice into a fine skill, where even subtle signs may alert the practitioner to a problem.

Visual information may be impaired if lighting is inadequate. Apart from the more obvious difficulties caused where lighting levels are low, shadows cast on to a part of the limb may adversely affect subjective aspects during biomechanical examination. Eyeballing describes a subjective visual technique that can be used to align joints before measurement, or to identify midpoints across skin surfaces as goniometric reference points. Passive examination of the subtalar joint range of motion and neutral position is considered to be an important element in understanding abnormal function of the foot. Inappropriate placement of reference lines, particularly on the curved surface of the back of the leg, is more likely to occur if one side of the leg is adequately lit and the other is not. A true vertical bisection of the leg may not be obtained. Consequently, the proportions of inversion and eversion contributing to the total range of motion, and determination of the neutral position, would be incorrect.

**Parallax error.** A potential source of measurement error, parallax error is particularly associated with joint position and movement. Parallax is an apparent difference in position or direction of an object caused by a change or relative change of observation point, as shown in Figure 4.3. Viewing an object or patient at right angles will eliminate parallax error. Measurement error will increase if the measurement instrument is not aligned with the plane of motion. A 90° alignment must also be ensured

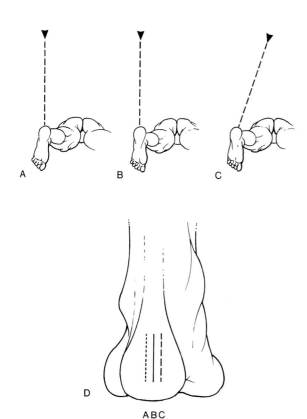

A    B    C

ABC

**Figure 4.3**  The effect of parallax on observation of the midpoint of the posterior aspect of the leg and heel **A.** Inappropriate positioning of the patient's leg leads to parallax error  **B.** With the patient's leg and the practitioner's eyes correctly aligned parallax error is eliminated  **C.** Inappropriate positioning of the practitioner's eyes leads to parallax error  **D.** The actual and apparent midpoints obtained from the relative eye and leg positions adopted in diagrams **A, B** and **C.**

when reading analogue measurement scales. Parallax error up to 3° was noted in one study (Griffith 1988).

The patient must be advised on the need for appropriate clothing if normal indoor dress inhibits a particular observation. Body parts must be clearly exposed where feasible. Shorts and a T-shirt, for example, allow a relatively uninhibited view of posture and movement.

### Touch

Touch involves many forms of direct and indirect (using instrumentation) physical contact with patients. During clinical examinations various components of the lower limb may be pushed, pulled, pressed, squeezed and twisted. The amount of force used is determined by feedback through the practitioner's proprioceptive pathways, the patient's response, sound and visual information. It is very subjective. The force used to test joint ranges of motion will need adjustment for different patients and different joints. Fluidity of the joints, muscle tone and the weight of the limb will all influence the force required to examine a joint effectively.

Instruments used in neurological and vascular assessments must be applied to the appropriate area and with an appropriate amount of force. Using neurotips, tuning forks and cotton wool requires a systematic approach and correct technique. For instance, inadvertently tickling the patient with cotton wool when testing for light touch will be interpreted through pain pathways rather than light touch receptors, invalidating the result.

Measurement of lower limb temperature can be obtained quantitatively with a digital thermometer, but most practitioners rely on touch. The practitioner's hand temperature will influence his appreciation of the patient's limb temperature. This can be demonstrated with a simple experiment. If both hands are inserted into a bowl of tepid water, having previously had one in cold and the other in hot, a clear difference in appreciation of temperature of the tepid water by each hand is noted. The subjective appreciation of temperature is therefore a relative phenomenon and a patient's limb will feel warmer to a practitioner with cold hands than one who has warm hands.

### Hearing

Doppler ultrasound units generate audible signals representing the velocity of blood flow. A normal arterial audio spectrum is triphasic, representing forward, reverse and forward blood flow. Considerable experience is necessary to develop the appropriate listening skills so that normal and abnormal sounds can be distinguished. However, artifacts can be produced if the application of the probe over the blood vessel is imprecise so that an artery and a vein are isonated simultaneously or the probe is not held steady. If the probe angle is incorrect the signal strength is reduced. A probe with an appropriate frequency must be selected, depending on the depth of the vessel of interest, so that adequate signal strength can be obtained. Connection to a computer with appropriate software enables the blood flow to be seen as a waveform providing a visual trace for interpretation (Fig. 4.4). Arterial and venous flows, pathological states and artifacts can be confirmed, with a permanent record produced for filing in case notes and inclusion in correspondence. Excellent accounts of the clinical use of Doppler ultrasound in the detection of peripheral vascular disease have been written by Vowden (1999), Grasty (1999) and Baker & Rayman (1999).

## The patient

The patient may be responsible for measurement errors for many reasons. General intelligence, mental disorder, anxiety, impaired hearing or sight or language difficulties could affect his ability to understand what is required. Patients may not follow instructions or respond appropriately or truthfully. They may be non-compliant. If the patient is anxious or annoyed, increased adrenaline (epinephrine) levels will elevate the basal metabolic rate, e.g. the pulse rate could be increased. Patients who are emotionally distressed may be less able to comply with the requirements of some types of measurement procedure.

It is not unusual for patients to find difficulty in relaxing during passive biomechanical measurements. Joint ranges and fluidity of motion can appear reduced. Forefoot varus or supinatus could be erroneously diagnosed if the patient fails to relax the tibialis anterior muscle, because contraction of this muscle inverts the forefoot relative to the hindfoot.

Neurological sensory tests may require a verbal response from the patient so that the result can be obtained. Assuming that the test is applied correctly, the patient must interpret the

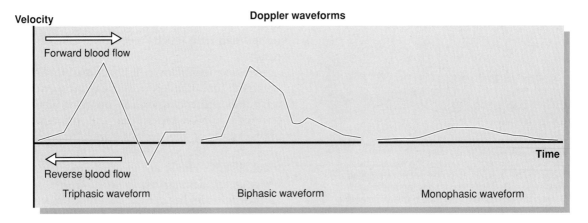

**Figure 4.4** Diagrammatic representations of Doppler output showing normal and abnormal waveforms (adapted from Baker & Rayman 1999).

> **Case history 5.4**
>
> A 65-year-old female patient attended the podiatry clinic complaining of weak muscles in her legs. She had noticed the weakness for some time, stating that if her symptoms continued to deteriorate she would have to give up her job as a school playground supervisor. Further questioning revealed that her weakness could more accurately be described as fatigue and heaviness of her legs walking to and from work. The patient had also noticed that climbing stairs brought upon a tight squeezing pain in her chest. Sitting down relieved the pain but prolonged sitting tended to make her ankles swell.
>
> **Diagnosis**: Congestive heart failure. This condition can have a direct effect upon the ability of the muscles to function under strain.

Rheumatic fever is a febrile disease occurring as a sequel to group A haemolytic streptococcal infections. It is characterised by inflammatory lesions of connective tissue structures, especially of the heart and blood vessels, and predisposes to bacterial endocarditis.

Having recorded disease states of which the patient is aware, enquire further about any systemic cardiovascular symptoms. Ask the patient if they:

- suffer from chest pains
- are ever short of breath
- experience palpitations
- find that their ankles swell
- are prone to fainting.

The most important cardiovascular symptom to elicit is chest pain because of the range of pathologies responsible for its occurrence. The differential diagnosis includes MI, angina pectoris, pneumonia, pericarditis and oesophageal reflux. The pain of angina is tight and pressure-like, precipitated by exercise and relieved by rest, and usually lasts for only a few minutes. The pain of an MI is similar in nature but is more intense, lasting from 30 minutes to 3 hours.

Dyspnoea (shortness of breath) may occur as a result of pulmonary oedema. In CHF there is an inadequacy in the supply of oxygenated blood. To compensate for this, first the heart rate

and then the volume of blood filling the left ventricle increases. Because it takes longer to fill the left ventricle, the pressure in the whole cardiac pulmonary system 'backs up', causing pulmonary congestion, reduced blood gas exchange and eventually pulmonary oedema. Pulmonary oedema and shortness of breath are, therefore, signs and symptoms of left-sided heart failure.

Right-sided heart failure is almost always associated with left-sided heart failure and gives rise to peripheral oedema. The right side of the heart can no longer deal with the volume of venous blood returning to the heart for transportation to the lungs and a 'back up' of pressure occurs in the systemic circulation, resulting in transudation of fluid into the peripheral connective tissue. Gravity will force most of the transudate to collect bilaterally in the feet and ankles. Initially, the patient will notice that the swelling reduces at night when the legs are recumbent. In chronic right-sided heart failure, the peripheral oedema will eventually be infiltrated by fibrous tissue that cannot be reduced by elevation.

Syncope (fainting) is a transient loss of consciousness. Cardiac disease such as arrhythmias and aortic stenosis can cause syncope by decreasing the cerebral blood supply. Other less-specific systemic cardiac symptoms include fatigue and decreased exertional tolerance.

To determine the presence of peripheral vascular disease the patient should be asked if they have ever had:

- a thrombosis or blood clot
- night cramps
- an ulcer on their leg or foot
- varicose veins and/or surgery.

Whereas cardiac problems may affect lower limb perfusion, peripheral vascular disease can occur in the absence of cardiac symptoms. The general enquiry may have already revealed sleeping problems, but the cardiovascular system investigation should determine whether sleep disturbance is due to cramping pain in the legs. Nocturnal cramps are a consequence of increased permeability of the microcirculation that accompanies the warming of the legs under bedding. In the presence of any impairment of the venous system, toxic metabolites will accumulate, increasing carbon dioxide tension while lowering oxygen levels. Muscle ischaemia follows, manifesting as a painful tautness of muscle fibre.

Also enquire further about any peripheral vascular symptoms. Ask the patient if they:

- get cramp at night
- get muscle cramps while walking
- suffer from chilblains
- notice their feet change colour if it is particularly cold.

All the above factors are signs and symptoms of peripheral vascular disease. Assessment of the vascular status of the lower limb is covered in detail in Chapter 6.

To determine the presence of haematological disease patients should be asked if they have:

- anaemia
- haemophilia
- any other blood disorder.

Haematological disorders should be considered. Anaemia occurs when red blood cells or haemoglobin content decreases because of blood loss, impaired production or excessive destruction of red blood cells. Tissue hypoxia results from anaemia and this in turn leads to cardiovascular and pulmonary compensations. Clinical symptoms depend upon the severity and duration of the anaemia. Severe anaemia is associated with weakness, vertigo, headaches, tiredness, gastrointestinal complaints and CHF.

Sickle cell disease is an inherited condition that can affect persons of African or West Indian descent. Those who inherit the gene from both patients have more than a 75% chance of developing the condition. Sickle cell individuals are prone to ulceration around the malleoli, a complaint more characteristic of older people with venous insufficiency. In most cases, patients will know whether they have sickle cell anaemia, as from early childhood the digits of the hands and feet tend to swell and are very painful. The use of tourniquets carries an increased risk of complication. A tourniquet causes relative anoxia and this in turn causes occlusion in small vessels due to changes in the haemodynamic qualities of red blood cells, which may lead to small vessel infarction and possibly digital gangrene.

## The respiratory system

To determine the presence of known systemic respiratory disease the patient should be asked if they have ever had (Table 5.3):

- asthma
- chronic bronchitis
- emphysema
- pulmonary embolism.

Asthma presents as a dry, wheezing cough accompanied by dyspnoea. Exercise, infection or

**Table 5.3** The clinical features and implications of respiratory diseases

| Disease | Clinical features | Clinical implications |
| --- | --- | --- |
| Asthma | Dyspnoea, wheezing, cough | Attacks may be provoked by exercise, infection or stress. May be treated with long-term corticosteroid therapy |
| Chronic bronchitis | Cough with expectoration of sputum for at least 3 months in 2 successive years | Commonly a history of cigarette smoking carries an accompanying risk of peripheral atherosclerosis |
| Emphysema | Dyspnoea with varying degrees of exertion | Sufferer will have limited exercise potential; in time will lead to right-sided heart failure and peripheral oedema |
| Pulmonary embolism | Pleuritic chest pain and haemoptysis | A life-threatening condition which may follow prolonged postoperative bed rest |

Inadequate levels of circulating thyroid hormone will lead to hypothyroidism. This condition may be discovered by asking the patient:

- Have you noticed any hair loss from your head or eyebrows?
- Are you troubled by dry scaly skin on your head or face?
- Have you noticed your hands or face getting puffy?
- Do you feel you have generally slowed down?
- Are you getting forgetful?
- Do you notice the cold?
- Has your weight increased?

In hypothyroidism the facial expression is dull and the features puffy with swelling around the eye sockets due to infiltration of mucopolysaccharides. The eyelids will droop due to decreased adrenergic drive and the skin and hair will be coarse and dry. The tongue may be enlarged, the voice hoarse and speech slow. Tarsal and carpal tunnel syndrome, caused by the infiltration of mucopolysaccharides, are common clinical features. Either form of thyroid disease renders the patient a poor candidate for foot surgery because it reduces his ability to deal with stress. Cardiac arrhythmias or metabolic imbalance may occur in stressful situations. Screening for thyroid disease is therefore essential and the above enquiry should be included in any presurgery assessment.

Disorders of the adrenal gland should also be considered. The adrenal gland has two functionally distinct parts, the cortex and the medulla. The more important of the two, the adrenal cortex, is essential for life as it produces glucocorticoids and mineralocorticoids, which are essential for maintaining blood volume during stress. The patient should be asked:

- Do you ever feel faint or dizzy when standing up after sitting for some time?
- Have you noticed any coloured patches or streaks developing on your skin?
- Have you had any problems with increased facial hair?
- Do you bruise easily?

The adrenal cortex is susceptible to either hypo- or hyperfunction. Hypofunction or Addison's disease is an autoimmune condition; the majority of clinical features are due to deficiency in glucocorticoid and mineralocorticoid (Table 5.9). The most relevant aspect of Addison's disease is the reduction in the level of cortisol. This hormone is normally produced in response to stress. Cortisol deficiency will reduce resistance to infection and trauma. Cushing's syndrome presents as an overproduction of glucocorticoids. High levels of cortisol increase carbohydrate production and lead to truncal obesity and development of a moon face. Purple striae or stretch marks will develop on the abdomen. An increased production of androgens may cause hirsutism. Thinning of the skin and increased risk of infection are important lower limb features of Cushing's disease. Osteoporosis may occur as a sequel to disruption of normal kidney function. Secondary diabetes mellitus may also occur as a sequel to Cushing's disease.

**Table 5.9**  Clinical features associated with disorders of the adrenal glands

| Disorder | Clinical features |
|---|---|
| Adrenal undersecretion (e.g. Addison's disease) | *Common features*: <br> Tiredness <br> Generalised weakness <br> Lethargy <br> Anorexia <br> Weight loss <br> Dizziness and postural hypotension <br> Pigmentation <br><br> *Less common features*: <br> Hypoglycaemia <br> Loss of body hair <br> Depression |
| Adrenal oversecretion (Cushing's syndrome) | Truncal obesity (moon face, buffalo hump, protuberant abdomen) <br> Thinning of skin <br> Purple striae <br> Excessive bruising <br> Hirsutism <br> Hypertension <br> Glucose intolerance <br> Muscle weakness and wasting, especially of proximal muscles <br> Back pain (osteoporosis and vertebral collapse) <br> Psychiatric disturbances |

Overactivity of the anterior pituitary gland will increase circulating levels of growth hormone, which results in excessive growth of feet, hands, jaw and soft tissue acromegaly. Excess growth hormone leads to glycogenesis: approximately 30% of acromegalics develop diabetes mellitus. Hypertension, due to inadequate renal clearance of phosphates, affects 30% of acromegalics. The majority of acromegalics suffer from constant headaches and joint pains. The condition, although rare, has significant foot health implications with a catalogue of signs and symptoms that will become apparent during virtually every stage of the functional enquiry.

## The locomotor system

To determine the presence of musculoskeletal disease the patient should be asked if they have ever had:

- any form of arthritis
- back, hip, knee, ankle or foot pain
- fractures of any bones in the legs or feet
- pulled or injured muscles in the legs
- joint swelling or stiffness
- limb pain during any specific activity.

The patient's account of spine or lower limb pain involving areas other than that of the presenting complaint should be obtained. The aim of the locomotor enquiry is to broaden the practitioner's outlook beyond the specific presenting complaint to a broader view of the locomotor system. Information from the locomotor enquiry will help to exclude conditions which may have

---

**Case history 5.10**

A 45-year-old female teacher presented with pain under the balls of both feet. She complained of general malaise and would go to bed much earlier in the evening than she used to. She described stiffness in her hands and knees, which was worse in the morning but improved after a hot bath and an aspirin. On examination the small joints of her hands and feet were swollen, leading the practitioner to suspect a systemic rather than local mechanical cause.
  **Diagnosis**: Rheumatoid arthritis. This was confirmed by a blood test, which showed a raised ESR (erylthrocyte sedimentation rate) and rheumatoid factor.

---

a systemic origin (Case history 5.10). Assessment of the locomotor system is considered in detail in Chapter 8.

## SUMMARY

Accurate diagnosis, which starts with taking the patient's medical and social history, forms the basis for formulation of an effective treatment plan. A format for history taking has been presented which covers all aspects of the patient's current and past medical status (Fig. 5.3). It has been emphasised that the personal social history is as important as the medical history, since it enables an assessment to be made about aspects of the patient's lifestyle which could influence any proposed treatment. The approach outlined in this chapter will ensure that a broad range of factors are taken into consideration when making a diagnosis and drawing up a treatment plan.

# 6

# Vascular assessment

*J. McLeod Roberts*

## INTRODUCTION

Assessment of the patient's vascular status is an essential part of the primary patient assessment. Davies & Horrocks (1992) noted that there has been an increase in the number of patients presenting with vascular disease. This chapter begins by explaining the purpose of a vascular assessment and then proceeds to provide an overview of the anatomy and physiology of the cardiovascular system. It continues by describing the necessary steps to be taken when assessing the cardiovascular and in particular the peripheral vascular status of the patient. Ranges of expected and abnormal values are included where appropriate. Simple, non-invasive tests are described which can be carried out by the practitioner using the minimum of equipment; hospital-based tests are also briefly described.

## THE PURPOSE OF A VASCULAR ASSESSMENT

The vascular status of the lower limb bears a direct relationship to tissue viability; furthermore, the severity of vascular disease has been shown to be associated with an increase in morbidity and mortality (Howell et al 1989). It will be apparent from this that assessment of the vascular status performs a useful screening function by detecting previously unidentified vascular abnormalities.

Information gained from a vascular assessment can be used to achieve the following:

- Identify whether the blood supply to and from the lower limb is adequate for normal function and tissue vitality.
- Identify vascular problems which could compromise the state of the tissues. It is important to detect not only the presence of such abnormalities but also the functional site, e.g. is it an arterial or venous insufficiency or a combination of both? These patients require monitoring so that complications – e.g. necrosis, ulceration and infection – can be prevented or their effects reduced.
- Identify whether there are any vascular abnormalities which could affect healing or the choice of treatment. These should be borne in mind when drawing up a treatment plan.

- Identify those patients in whom vascular conditions require further investigation by referral to a specialist.

# OVERVIEW OF THE CARDIOVASCULAR SYSTEM

## ANATOMY OF THE CARDIOVASCULAR SYSTEM

The cardiovascular system (CVS) consists of a closed system of vessels through which blood and lymph are pumped around the body by means of the heart (Fig. 6.1).

### The heart

The heart is constructed as a double pump in series: one pump comprising the left side of the

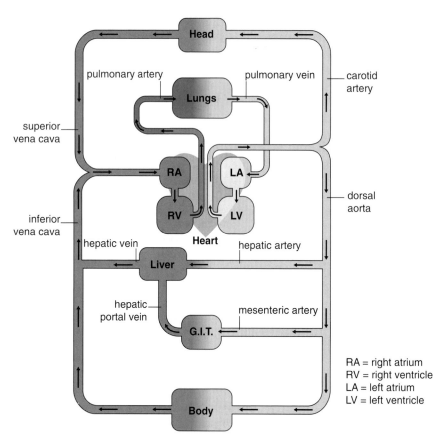

**Figure 6.1** The major vessels of the cardiovascular system. In the body proper, the dorsal aorta and the vena cavae run in the central axis, but for purposes of clarity they are shown to the right and left of the body, respectively. RA = right atrium, RV = right ventricle, LA = left atrium, LV = left ventricle, GIT = gastrointestinal tract.

RA = right atrium
RV = right ventricle
LA = left atrium
LV = left ventricle

heart and the other the right side (Fig. 6.2). Each pump has two chambers. Each upper chamber or atrium is a receiving vessel with a thin muscle wall or myocardium, whereas the lower chambers or ventricles are the dispersing vessels and therefore have much thicker muscle walls to generate strong propulsive forces (Fig. 6.3). The heart is lined by endocardium and surrounded by a tough, non-extensible pericardium. The endocardium forms the cusps of one-way valves, called the tricuspid and bicuspid valves, which control the flow of blood through the heart. It also forms semilunar valves, which control the entry of blood into the vessels leaving the heart. Closure of these valves is responsible for the two heart sounds, 'lub-dup', which can be heard through a stethoscope applied to the chest wall.

The heart serves two circulations. The right ventricle serves the pulmonary or minor circulation and sends deoxygenated blood via the pulmonary arteries to the lungs, whereas the left ventricle supplies the systemic or major circulation with oxygenated blood through the aorta to the body (Fig. 6.2). Oxygenated blood is returned from the lungs via the right and left pulmonary veins into the left atrium and deoxygenated

blood from the body flows through the superior and inferior vena cavae into the right atrium.

## Peripheral circulation

The blood flows through the two circulations via a system of vessels of varying diameters (Table 6.1).

### Arterial tree

The vessels which transport blood to the tissues are called arteries. These branch into consecutively smaller vessels called arterioles. The walls of arteries consist of three layers – the tunica intima, tunica media and tunica adventitia – all of which are lined with vascular endothelium, whose cells secrete a variety of substances essential for maintenance of vessel wall and circulatory function (Fig. 6.4A). All the vessels have some smooth muscle in the tunica media to enable them to change diameter, but arterioles have the greater proportion. The arteries leaving the heart have a high proportion of elastic tissue in their walls, which enables them to act as secondary pumps, whereas the rest of the arterial tree consists of muscular distributing vessels. The smallest arterioles deliver blood to capillary beds.

### Venous tree

Blood is drained from the tissue beds by small vessels called venules, which join to form larger vessels called veins. The three layers seen in the arterial walls are again present but the proportions differ, as can be seen in Figure 6.4A. The vascular endothelium forms semilunar valves in the veins and venules to prevent backflow of

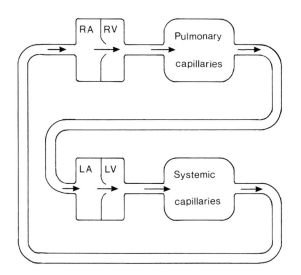

**Figure 6.2**  The heart is a double pump in series. It serves two circulations, the low-pressure pulmonary and the high-pressure systemic circulation.

**Table 6.1**  The anatomy of peripheral vessels

| Vessel | Diameter | Wall thickness |
| --- | --- | --- |
| Aorta | 25 cm | 2 mm |
| Artery | 4 mm | 1 mm |
| Arteriole | 30 µm | 20 µm |
| Capillary | 6 µm | 1 µm |
| Venule | 20 µm | 2 µm |
| Vein | 5 mm | 500 µm |
| Vena cava | 30 mm | 1.5 mm |

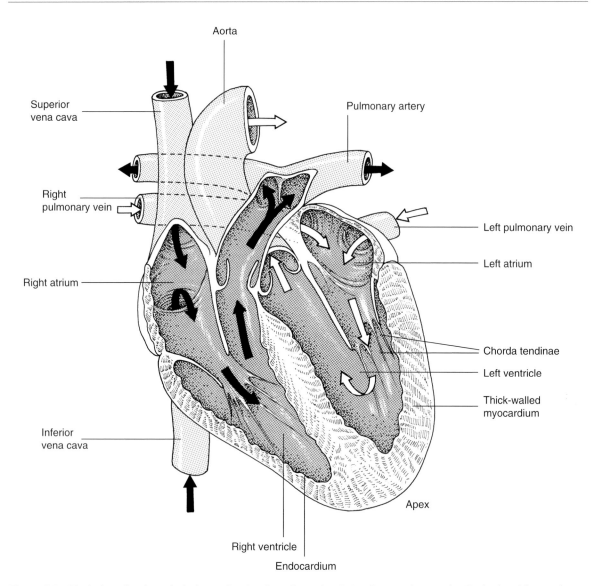

**Figure 6.3** Vertical section through the heart showing the valves, chorda tendinae, main vessels attached and the varying thickness of the myocardium. The direction of flow of oxygenated (non-shaded arrows) and deoxygenated (shaded arrows) blood is also shown.

blood. Veins are found either in the superficial fascia or deep in the muscle. Communicating veins link the two types so that blood can drain from the superficial veins to the deep ones.

### Capillary

A third type of vessel, the capillary, links arterioles and venules. This is the smallest and most numerous vessel, having only a thin-walled endothelium (Fig. 6.4B). It permeates all the tissue beds so that no tissue cell is far from a capillary. Flow of blood into individual capillaries is regulated by smooth muscle sphincters in vessels called metarterioles, which are situated at the entrances to the capillaries. Capillaries can be bypassed by arteriovenous (A-V) anastomoses: these are vessels which form a direct link

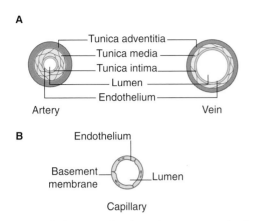

**A**

Artery — Vein
- Tunica adventitia
- Tunica media
- Tunica intima
- Lumen
- Endothelium

**B**

Capillary
- Endothelium
- Basement membrane
- Lumen

**Figure 6.4  A.** Cross-section through an artery and vein showing tunica intima, media and adventitia  **B.** Cross-section through a capillary. Note the relative proportions of thickness in artery and vein and its absence in the capillary.

between an arteriole and a venule (Fig. 6.5A). In peripheral cutaneous sites exposed to extremes of temperature, such as the skin of fingertips, apices of toes, nose and earlobes, the A-V anastomoses are very numerous and form specialised structures under the nail beds called glomus bodies or Sucquet–Hoyer canals (Fig. 6.5B).

*Microcirculation*

The smaller-diameter vessels collectively form the microcirculation.

*Collaterals*

Most microcirculations are served by more than one branch of the arterial tree. These parallel

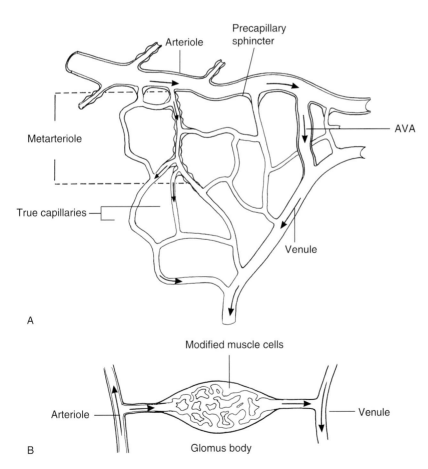

**Figure 6.5  A.** Diagram of the microcirculation showing an arteriole and a venule connected by an arteriovenous anastomosis (AVA) and a capillary network. The AVA is a shorter, tortuous, muscular vessel of a larger calibre. The capillary network comprises metarterioles, which have a muscular coat, and the distal portion of the capillary network, which consists solely of endothelial cells  **B.** Diagram showing the specialised AVA under the nail bed (glomus body).

branches are called collaterals and may anastomose freely or hardly at all, the degree of communication varying from tissue to tissue (Fig. 6.6A). The lack of anastomoses in the coronary circulation is responsible for the dramatic effects of an occlusion in the left coronary artery (Fig. 6.6B).

## Lymphatic tree

Lymphatic vessels are very similar in structure to veins and capillaries, except that the smallest vessels are blind-ended (Fig. 6.7). They drain the tissues and transport lymph through various lymph nodes, eventually rejoining the peripheral circulation through the thoracic duct.

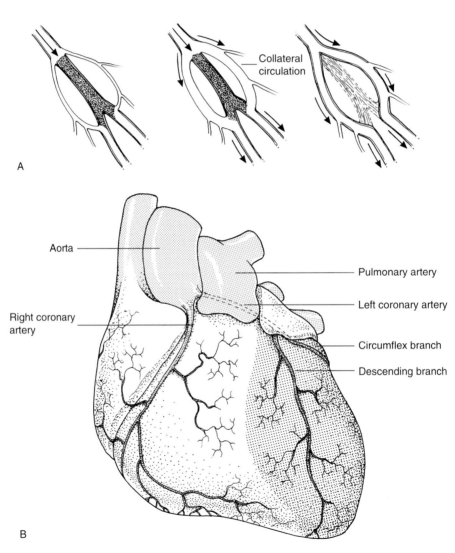

**Figure 6.6   A.** Small side vessels normally carry an insignificant fraction of blood into the peripheral tissues. Damage or occlusion of the major arteries alters pressure relationships to divert blood through the side vessels (collateral circulation). **B.** Anterior view of heart showing lack of anastomoses between arterial vessels supplying the myocardium. Left coronary artery supplies hatched area, right coronary artery supplies unhatched area. The lack of anastomoses between left and right coronary arteries explains why an occlusion of the left coronary artery can be so catastrophic.

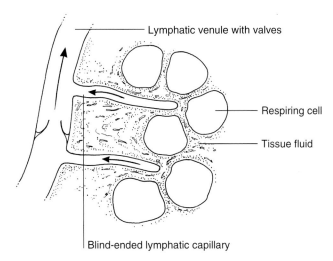

Lymphatic venule with valves

Respiring cell

Tissue fluid

Blind-ended lymphatic capillary

**Figure 6.7** Diagram showing a blind-ended lymphatic capillary.

*Tissue fluid*

While capillaries bring blood close to all body cells, a diffusion medium is needed to enable nutrients, waste products and gases to be exchanged between the cells and the blood and lymph. This medium is tissue fluid, which is continuously forming from blood at capillary and postcapillary venular sites as a result of hydrostatic and oncotic pressures (Fig. 6.8). Some tissue fluid is reabsorbed back into these vessels, the remainder draining into the lymphatic capillaries to be returned to the general circulation.

## NORMAL PHYSIOLOGY OF THE CARDIOVASCULAR SYSTEM

The essential function of the CVS is to ensure that there is sufficient perfusion pressure to maintain, under all circumstances, an adequate flow of blood to the vital organs, especially the brain. This is achieved by alteration of the rate and force of contraction of the myocardium and by varying the diameter throughout the peripheral circulation. In periods of increased demand, non-vital areas will have a reduced flow and this may very well affect the lower limb.

The heart contracts about once every 0.8 seconds in a healthy resting adult. The heart beat is divided into two phases: the relaxation phase or diastole and the contraction phase or systole. Systole is the shorter of the two phases, lasting about 0.3 seconds, though with increased heart rate, the period of diastole shortens.

The volume of blood ejected from each ventricle is the same and is called the stroke volume. In a healthy resting adult about 70 ml is ejected at each contraction of the ventricle. Since the normal resting heart rate is an average of 72 beats per minute, the volume ejected from each ventricle in 1 minute is approximately 5 litres and is known as the cardiac output.

The myocardium has the ability to contract without nerve impulses. This property is called myogenicity and is due to the presence of specialised 'pacemaker' cells which generate spontaneous action potentials. The most important of these is the sinoatrial (SA) node, situated in the right atrium (Fig. 6.9). The action potential spreads rapidly through the other specialised conducting tissues and then out over the rest of the myocardium through gap junctions between the cells. This ensures that the cells can respond as a unit, producing a coordinated wave of contraction which pushes the blood in the desired direction. Apart from these specialised pathways, the septa that divide the four chambers of the heart consist of fibrous, non-conducting tissue.

While the heart can contract without nervous stimulation, it is essential that it can alter its activity according to the differing demands placed upon it as mentioned earlier. One way that this is achieved is via the autonomic system (ANS) (Ch. 7). The two branches of the ANS send fibres to the SA node. The sympathetic nerve acts on the heart via specific receptors called $beta_1$-receptors, the action of which is to increase cardiac output by increasing both stroke volume (positive inotropy) and heart rate (positive chronotropy). The parasympathetic nerve to the heart is called the vagus and causes slowing of

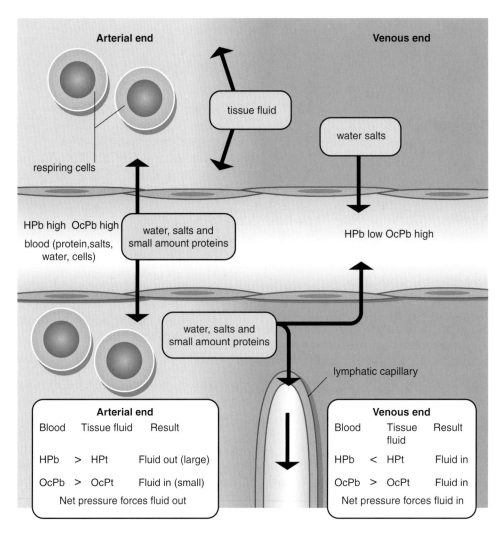

HPb(t) = hydrostatic pressure of blood (and pressure flow)
OcPb(t) = oncolic pressure of blood (b) and tissue fluid (t)
oncolic pressure = oncolic pressure due to protein

**Figure 6.8**   The process of formation and reabsorption of tissue fluid in an ideal capillary. Movement of fluid in and out of the capillary will vary according to the precise balance of pressures along the capillary at any one time.

HDLC <35 mg/dl (0.9 mmol/l) are considered in the United States to have subclinical CAD (Hecht & Superko 2001).

**Coronary angiography.** This involves introduction of a diagnostic catheter through the femoral artery into the left ventricle and associated vessels (Kumar & Clark 1990c). Pressures in various of the heart chambers and main vessels can be measured directly. Blood samples can be taken to measure oxygen content and ischaemic metabolites such as lactate and contrast cine-angiograms can be taken by injection of a radio-opaque dye at the site to be investigated. Digital subtraction angiography produces better-quality angiograms.

**Myocardial perfusion scintigraphy (radionuclide perfusion imaging).** This is a very sensitive test using exercise thallium-201 or technetium-99m imaging to detect coronary artery disease (Kapoor & Singh 1993b, Kumar & Clark 1990d).

## PERIPHERAL VASCULAR SYSTEM

It is important to distinguish between an impoverished arterial supply, reduced venous drainage and impaired lymphatic drainage, though of course more than one impairment may coexist.

## ARTERIAL INSUFFICIENCY

### Medical history

Conditions which can affect the arterial supply to the lower limb can be divided into those that lead to acute and those that lead to chronic problems (Table 6.3).

Most arterial problems affecting the lower limb are chronic in nature, leading to peripheral arterial occlusive disease (PAOD) and resulting in ischaemia and poor tissue viability. The most common cause of PAOD, which is also called peripheral vascular disease (PVD), is atherosclerosis. This is a pathological process involving formation of a fatty plaque or atheroma in the intima of large and medium-sized arteries (Murphie 2001a). The atheroma itself causes no obstruction to blood flow, but its tendency to ulcerate promotes thrombus formation, which

**Table 6.3**   Causes of arterial insufficiency in the foot

| Acute | Extrinsic: |
|---|---|
| | light clothing |
| | tourniquet |
| | plaster cast |
| | trauma |
| | frostbite |
| | immersion foot |
| | Intrinsic: |
| | thrombosis |
| | embolus |
| | ruptured aneurysm |
| | oedema |
| Transient | (usually lead to acute problems but may progress to chronic) |
| | Raynaud's phenomenon |
| | Chilblains |
| | Hereditary cold fingers |
| Chronic | Atherosclerosis |
| | Vasculitis |
| | Thromboangiitis obliterans (Buerger's disease) |
| | Arteriolosclerosis? |

causes narrowing (stenosis) or complete occlusion of the vessel. In addition, the thrombus is likely to embolise and be swept away to cause obstruction further down the arterial tree. There appears to be little evidence to suggest, as was previously believed, that a similar process occurs in the micro-circulation (Murphie 2001b). Although hyalinisation (arteriolosclerosis) and thickening of basement membranes and functional abnormalities of small vessels have been observed, these changes occur mainly in renal and retinal vessels, and are not considered to have major effects on the vascular status of the foot. Such changes mainly affect people with diabetes, but not exclusively. Much less common causes of PAOD are vasculitis, thromboangiitis obliterans and arterial emboli. Vasculitis is inflammation of blood vessels seen in a large number of rheumatic and connective tissue diseases. Any vessel can be affected, with the most serious consequences being in the arterial tree, resulting in partial or total occlusion.

Some of the conditions associated with vasculitis are:

- rheumatoid arthritis
- systemic lupus erythematosus (SLE)
- polymyositis

- dermatomyositis
- systemic sclerosis
- polyarteritis nodosa
- giant-cell arteritis
- erythema nodosum
- Henoch–Schönlein syndrome.

Thromboangiitis obliterans is characterised by inflammatory changes in small and medium-sized arteries and veins. It mainly affects young males and there is a very strong association with smoking. All signs and symptoms of arterial ischaemia and superficial phlebitis of the hands and feet may be present. Eventually, distal necrosis occurs.

Arterial emboli can be composed of any obstructive body that lodges in the smaller vessels of the arterial tree, causing ischaemia distally. The most common embolus is formed by fragmentation of a thrombus, such as a mural thrombus found on the endocardium, especially around the heart valves, or in the arteries, mostly at sites of bifurcation, where turbulence is most likely. Emboli may occlude arterioles and capillaries, causing isolated patches of digital necrosis. The source of such emboli may be septic thrombus from infection or deformed red blood cells as seen in sickle cell anaemia. Any history of previous MI, stroke or transient ischaemic attacks suggests the presence of atherosclerosis which, in addition to affecting the coronary and cerebral arteries, may also be affecting the arterial supply to the lower limb. A past history of vascular surgery such as coronary or femoropopliteal bypass grafting is also a good indicator that atherosclerosis may be present. A history of cryovascular disorders (e.g. chilblains, Raynaud's disease/phenomenon) should be noted as the attacks of vasospasm may become chronic and cause painful digital ulceration. (Case history 6.2).

## Symptoms

Inadequate blood supply to the lower limb leads to a range of signs and symptoms that are known as the six Ps:

- pain

---

**Case history 6.2**

A 35-year-old female Caucasian first presented to the clinic when aged 24, complaining of broken skin on the toes. The patient presently lived alone as she had recently separated from her partner and she had a history of poor circulation to both hands and feet. Footwear was inadequate for winter, and foot hygiene was poor. Examination of the lower limbs revealed pale skin and cold feet. The lesser toes were held in flexion deformities. No hairs were present. The nail on the left fifth toe was black. The skin was tight, shiny and smooth. There were small, painful ulcers on the apices of toes and fingers. All ulcers showed signs of infection. Pedal pulses were palpable but feeble. Popliteal pulses were stronger. Ankle–brachial pressure indices at the dorsalis pedis artery for right and left foot were 1.0 and 0.97, respectively. There was no evidence of underlying systemic disease.

A diagnosis of idiopathic Raynaud's disease was made. The condition was exacerbated by personal and social factors. The repeated breakdown of lesions, as detailed in the patient's record over the past 4 years, was due to the underlying vasospastic disorder, which was worsened by cold weather, self-neglect and emotional upsets. Current treatment was successful in healing the lesions but without continued patient compliance the overall prognosis is poor.

---

- pallor
- pulselessness
- paraesthesia
- paralysis
- perishing cold.

Pain is usually associated with arterial insufficiency. It is important that the site, nature, duration and aggravating factors of the pain are recorded. This information can be very helpful when assessing the prognosis of diseases that affect the arterial supply. Inadequate blood supply to respiring tissues may be an acute situation, producing a characteristic range of signs and symptoms, including pain, pallor and lack of pulses. When the deficiency is prolonged, the tissues eventually suffer irreversible damage and this stage can be recognised by mottling, muscle tenderness, motor or sensory deficit and necrosis. Continuation of the condition will lead to a chronic state of insufficiency, accompanied by pain on exercise, or even at rest if very severe, and necrosis and ulceration. The following types

**Table 6.4** The Fontaine classification of peripheral vascular disease (PVD)

| Stage | Symptoms |
| --- | --- |
| 1 | Occlusive arterial disease but no symptoms (due to collaterals) |
| 2 | Intermittent claudication |
| 3 | Ischaemic rest pain (usually worse at night, relieved by dependency) |
| 4 | Severe rest pain with ulceration/necrosis (gangrene) |

of ischaemic pain can occur and lead to the Fontaine classification of PVD (Table 6.4).

### Intermittent claudication

Just as angina pectoris indicates insufficient blood supply to the myocardium, so intermittent claudication indicates inadequate blood supply to the periphery. When the blood supply is inadequate, the deficiency will be accentuated on exercise. The exercising muscles have to respire anaerobically and produce metabolites which are not cleared by the blood. These cause ischaemic pain, which forces the patient to stop the activity. Resting for a few minutes reduces the amount of metabolites produced and allows the patient to continue walking for a further period. The distance walked before onset of the pain is called the ischaemic or claudication distance and is a good indication of the severity of the condition. The exercise should be standardised, e.g. 4 minutes at 0% incline at 4 km/h (Lainge & Greenhalgh 1980). The site of the ischaemic pain is an indication of the site of the occlusion. It should be borne in mind, however, that patients with neuropathy may not complain of intermittent claudication.

### Night cramps

If the blood supply is more severely compromised, the patient will experience night cramps, which are alleviated by dangling the legs over the side of the bed or walking on a cool floor. The warmth of the bedclothes increases the metabolic rate of the tissues and so increases their demand for oxygen; this cannot be met and produces ischaemic pain. Using gravity to

aid flow and cooling the limb helps to reduce metabolic activity.

### Rest pain

This is the most severe condition of critical limb ischaemia. Here the blood supply is inadequate even at rest, walking is impossible and the only way that the peripheral tissues can obtain any blood is by gravity. The legs must always lie below the level of the heart, either by raising the head of the bed or by sleeping in a chair. Even contact of the bedclothes on the limbs may be too painful. Cages are sometimes used to protect the limbs.

## Observation

While an experienced practitioner can glean considerable information from simple observation, it is important not to rely on these observations alone, but to view them as part of the whole picture. The patient should be seated on a couch in a comfortably warm room.

### Colour

Table 6.5 shows the range of colour changes seen in the lower limb and their significance.

### Tissue viability

**Hairs.** A poor blood supply leads to inadequate nourishment for skin and soft tissues. The skin will appear thin, shiny, and dry with absent hairs (Plate 1). Friction from boots and depilatories could be less worrying causes.

**Atrophy.** In chronic situations atrophy (wastage) of soft tissue, including muscle, will also be present. This is especially noticeable on the plantar surface of the foot. In severe limb ischaemia, muscle tone will be lost and the limb will appear lifeless.

### Ischaemic ulcers

An impaired peripheral circulation makes ulcers more likely to develop as the tissues are unable to

**Table 6.5** Interpretation of colour changes in the lower limb

| Colour | Causes |
| --- | --- |
| Pink | Healthy circulation |
| White/pale | Cold, anaemia, chilblains, Raynaud's phenomenon, cardiac failure |
| White below demarcation line | Severe ischaemia |
| Blue (peripheral cyanosis) | Cold, chilblains, Raynaud's phenomenon, venous stasis |
| Blue seen with central cyanosis | Cardiac/respiratory failure |
| Hazy blue | Infection, necrosis |
| Red | Heat, exercise, extreme cold (cold-induced vasodilation), inflammation, infection (cellulitis), chilblains, Raynaud's phenomenon |
| Brown | Haemosiderosis, moist necrosis |
| Black | Bruise, shoe dye, necrosis |

withstand the normal daily stresses on the lower limb. The characteristics of the lesion can assist in diagnosis of the circulatory problem, since ulcers caused by ischaemia differ in many respects from those caused by other deficiencies such as poor drainage or neuropathy (Ch. 17). Ischaemic ulcers are caused by trauma and are usually very painful, unless there is neuropathy present, as for example in some diabetic patients. There is lack of granulation tissue and low amounts of exudate, but slough is often present. The borders are well demarcated and they may have a 'punched out' appearance (Plate 2). They often occur first under the toe nails, on the apices of the toes or around the borders of the feet, a contributory factor usually being tight or ill-fitting footwear. Leg elevation can exacerbate the pain, whereas lowering the leg into dependency can improve the blood supply and ease the pain. Ischaemic ulcers are unlikely to heal unless there is an improvement in blood supply. Ulcers of any type are less likely to heal if the patient is on medication which reduces cardiac output, e.g. beta-blockers.

### Nails

Poor blood supply will affect the nails. These may be crumbly, discoloured or thickened. They are prone to fungal infection and pitting. The latter should be differentially diagnosed from dermatological conditions such as psoriasis (Ch. 9).

### Necrosis (gangrene)

Severe ischaemia, if unrelieved, will progress to necrosis or dry gangrene, with the most distal regions being affected first. The tissue will appear hard, black and mummified, with a clear demarcation line between dead and living tissue (Plate 3). Ulceration and infection may cause a septic vasculitis, which again leads to ischaemia and necrosis, but here the tissue remains moist and usually has a distinctive smell. This is wet gangrene. Pus and infection of surrounding tissue is present. The presence of proximal arterial occlusion and poor collateral development may be contributing factors.

### Oedema

Oedema is not usually associated with poor peripheral arterial supply. If present bilaterally, the cause is likely to be a central one such as congestive heart failure. Unilateral or localised oedema may be due to infection, trauma, allergy or impaired venous or lymphatic drainage (Table 6.6).

## Clinical tests

The following tests should be repeated for both lower limbs and require none or very simple apparatus of the type usually found in a practitioner's clinical environment. Again some of these tests are of greater significance than others in aiding diagnosis.

### Temperature gradient

The back of the practitioner's hand should be used to stroke the anterior surface of the patient's

waveform indicates disease (Fig. 6.13B), although a diphasic response can be seen with ageing as the vessels lose compliability (Case history 6.3). Forward and reverse flow simultaneously suggests turbulence, as would occur just distal to a site of stenosis. A monophasic response always indicates disease, but care must be taken first to ensure that the technique is not at fault. Patients with bradycardia will have a weak triphasic sound and patients with tachycardia will show only a biphasic sound as the heart is beating too rapidly for reverse flow to occur. The amplitude of the waveform is not significant since it depends on the angle of the probe.

### Claudication distance

If the patient complains of intermittent claudication or if pedal pulses seem weak or absent, this test can be used to give an indication of the severity of the arterial occlusion. The patient is exercised, preferably on a treadmill, as the exercise should be standardised, and the distance the patient walks before the onset of pain is noted. The treadmill should be at 0% incline and at a speed of 4 km/h. No patient should be exercised if there is a history of angina and it is recommended that a full resuscitation kit should always be present for any exercise test.

### Ankle–brachial pressure index (ABPI)

This was first described by Yao in the 1960s. The ankle–brachial index provides a good indication of the presence of ischaemia in the lower limb. It can be used quantitatively since it also correlates well with the patient's symptoms, walking distance and angiography. It can be used to determine the optimum level of amputation and prognoses for grafts (Ameli et al 1989, Davies 1992).

The ankle–brachial pressure index is arrived at by recording the systolic pressure at the brachial artery and at the posterior tibial artery (ankle). Practitioners may find Doppler easier to use than a stethoscope when trying to take a reading of the systolic pressure in lower limb arteries. The reading obtained for the ankle is then divided by the brachial systolic reading and is expressed as a ratio. The value obtained at the ankle will depend on the position of the patient. If the person is supine and the legs are at the same horizontal level as the heart the ratio should be 1. If the person is sitting or standing, the pressure in the artery at the ankle will be greater than in the arm, because of the vertical column of blood between heart and ankle. As a rule of thumb the ankle systolic pressure will be 2 mmHg higher for every inch below the heart. Thus the ratio will be greater than 1. Average

---

**Case history 6.3**

A 59-year-old female Caucasian presented to the clinic with an ulcer of 12 months' duration over the right medial maleolus. The patient complained that the skin had been itchy prior to the ulcer occurring and had developed following a knock to the right ankle. Pain was worsened on standing for long periods and relieved by elevation of the legs. She had no symptoms of paraesthesia or claudication. Examination of the lower limbs was remarkable for pitting oedema, varicose veins, haemosiderosis, atrophe blanche and gravitational eczema in the distal third of the right limb. The skin was warm, pedal pulses were bounding and regular (70 beats per minute) in the left foot but pedal pulses in the right foot could not be palpated because of the oedema. Both right pedal pulses were located with Doppler and gave a regular, biphasic signal. There was no evidence of trophic changes to skin or soft tissue. An ischaemic (ankle–brachial) index was not undertaken on the right leg

because of the ulceration present. The ischaemic index for the left leg was 1.2. The Doppler signal of the popliteal vein in the popliteal fossa indicated venous reflux.

The past medical history revealed that the patient had suffered a deep vein thrombosis while recuperating from a major abdominal operation when 20 years old. The thrombosis had been treated effectively at the time but the patient had noticed some 10 years later that her right leg began to ache and feel heavy after prolonged standing. When she was about 40 years old her ankle started to swell towards the end of the day and by the time she was 50 the skin around the area had become discoloured and itchy. Despite a range of treatments the ulcer had not healed.

A diagnosis was made of venous ulceration, as a result of post-thrombotic complications. These ulcers are notoriously difficult to heal and account for the majority of lower limb ulceration.

values for healthy adults in the sitting position are 0.98–1.31 (Davies 1992).

A ratio which is greater than 1 does not always mean that all is well. Elderly patients may show calcification of the tunica media of muscular arteries (Mönckeberg's sclerosis) which, although independent of any atherosclerotic process and clinically insignificant, leads to incompressibility and a false high systolic pressure value. People with diabetes are also prone to calcification of the artery wall (not to be confused with Mönckeberg's sclerosis), again leading to incompressibility of the artery. Nevertheless, 'the measurement of ankle pressure using Doppler is the single most valuable adjunct to the assessment of the blood supply to the foot' (Faris 1991).

Any value below 1 should be checked again. Values less than 0.8 suggest some obstruction in the more proximal part of the artery to the lower limb, although it is possible to find no associated lesions in such patients. Values of 0.75 or less indicate severe problems, and at values below 0.5 healing is unlikely to take place, the leg being in a pre-necrotic state. Critical limb ischaemia is said to be present when the ankle systolic pressure falls below 50 mmHg or the toe systolic pressure falls below 30 mmHg (Lowe 1993). Ischaemic ulcers may be present.

If severe ischaemia is suspected, but a high ABPI is obtained due to calcification, the Pole test can be used to calculate the ABPI (Smith et al 1994). The Pole test is a variation on the Buerger test using a mini-Doppler machine. With the patient supine, the suspected pedal artery is located and the affected leg raised until the pulse can no longer be heard. The vertical distance between the heart and this point is noted. Ankle systolic pressure is calculated using the formula 13 cm = 10 mmHg. Values of less than 40 cm (31 mmHg) suggest severe occlusion. Calcification will have no effect on this reading, but the method is limited to those patients with pressures less than 60 mmHg. It is also worth remembering that the peroneal artery is usually spared from calcification.

Since mild to moderate atherosclerotic change may not affect the resting ABPI the effects of exercise on the index are often observed (Davies 1992). Again a standardised treadmill exercise should be used (4 km/h, 0% incline, 4 minutes). In a healthy adult, unless exercise is severe, the index will show no change or will rise but rapidly returns to resting value once exercise has stopped. In a person suffering from peripheral vascular disease, the index will not rise and may fall, taking a long time to return to resting values. Heavy exercise may produce a fall in the index in healthy subjects due to shunting of blood from the distal arteries to the exercising muscles.

If the patient cannot be exercised, the hyperaemic test can be used. A second occlusion cuff is placed proximal to the first and inflated to above the systolic pressure for 2 minutes or as long as the presence of ischaemic pain will allow. It is then deflated and the systolic blood pressure is immediately taken. The second cuff occludes the arterial supply. Since venous drainage is also temporarily interrupted, metabolites will accumulate in the area. These have a vasodilatory effect on the blood vessels, so that in a healthy person, on releasing the second cuff, blood will rush into the area, producing a temporary hyperaemia. This will cause a slight rise in systolic blood pressure and so raise the value of the ABPI, but will quickly return to normal values. In a patient with peripheral vascular disease the narrowed arteries will be unable to respond to the vasodilatory effects of the metabolites, either because they are unable to dilate or because the occlusion prevents an increased flow, so that the ABPI will either stay the same or fall.

If a low ankle–brachial index is recorded, the index should be calculated at progressively higher positions up the leg, to ascertain the site of the occlusion. When using the ankle–brachial pressure index it is also important to remember that the value obtained for the ankle cannot accurately predict the healing of lesions in the forefoot although pedal arteries are rarely affected by atherosclerosis. Digital cuffs can be used to assess the systolic reading in toes. A Doppler head of 10 mHz is preferable although not essential. ABPI of the peroneal nerve, toe pressures and analysis of the Doppler waveform will give a reliable indication of the presence of significant ischaemia, which will be revealed as reduced

ABPI, reduced toe pressure and dampening of the Doppler waveform.

The cardinal signs of ischaemia can be summarised as follows:

- diminished or absent pedal pulses
- ABPI <0.9
- ischaemic pain.

## Hospital tests

If an ischaemic limb has been identified, further investigation may be required to assess:

- suitability for reconstructive surgery
- the prognosis for the healing of ulcers
- the level at which amputations should be performed.

### *Macrocirculation*

**Duplex ultrasound.** This combines B mode ultrasound and Doppler to give both an image of the artery under investigation and the flow within that artery (Banga 1995). It takes time and requires a level of expertise, but using Doppler and pulse-generated run-off (PGR) a complete non-invasive assessment of the lower limb can be achieved, which reduces the need for contrast angiography.

**Angiography (arteriography).** At present this procedure, especially using intra-arterial digital subtraction angiography, remains the gold standard for imaging the arterial supply of the lower limb. A needle is inserted into the femoral artery and a radio-opaque dye is injected just proximal to the occlusion. It can be used to locate occlusions and stenotic vessels and to determine whether a collateral circulation has been established. It is used to help determine the most appropriate revascularisation procedure and, if a bypass procedure is to be performed, the site of the distal anastomosis. It also is used to predict the prognosis for limb salvage and graft patency. It can also be used during surgery, to enable the surgeon to have an accurate picture of distal run-off. Being an invasive procedure, it carries more risks than non-invasive procedures, which are likely to replace it as technicalities improve.

**Magnetic resonance imaging (MRI) and positron emission tomography (PET) scanning.** These are expensive, more recent procedures which can be used to visualise the various parts of the circulation. Initially, doubts were raised as to the value of such procedures in the absence of evidence to suggest any improvement in patient outcome (Kapoor & Singh 1993c) but recent improvements in resolution using gadolinium enhancement now enable imaging of digital vessels as small as 1 mm diameter and have led Mercer & Berridge (2000) to consider magnetic resonance angiography as the modality of the future, eventually replacing contrast angiography.

### *Microcirculation*

**Capillaroscopy.** With the patient in a sitting position, the capillaries of the pedal nail fold can be examined, using an oil immersion microscope under a strong light. The nutritive capillaries are distinct and well filled with blood in a person with no arterial disease but, as ischaemia progresses, the capillaries become hazy and less distinct. Capillaroscopy can be used to predict those patients likely to develop critical limb ischaemia as well as the likelihood of healing of ischaemic ulcers.

**Transcutaneous oxygen tension (TcpO$_2$).** The skin is heated to arterialise the capillaries and the oxygen which diffuses to the surface of the skin equilibrates with an electrolyte solution held in a small chamber on the skin. The partial pressure of oxygen in the solution is measured by an electrode which screws into the chamber. This value reflects the difference between oxygen supply and consumption in the local tissues. Severe ischaemia is indicated if the value is below 40 mmHg, when healing will be unlikely. This is not a routine test but can be used as a predictor of level of amputation and of the success of angioplasty.

**Photoelectric plethysmography.** This method is used to measure skin blood pressure. A light-emitting diode is placed on the skin and a photocell is used to detect the emitted light, which is proportional to the amount of haemoglobin in the tissues. A sphygmomanometer cuff is used to blanch the skin. The cuff is then slowly deflated and the pressure point at which a flow signal returns is taken to be the skin perfusion pressure. A similar piece of apparatus is used to measure oxygen percentage saturation of the blood in pulse oximetry (Coull 1988).

**Isotope clearance.** This method is used to measure skin perfusion pressure (SPP) and skin vascular resistance (SVR) in the compromised foot in order to ascertain the likelihood of the healing of ischaemic ulcers. The SVR can be calculated from the graph of clearance values and applied pressure. A straight-line relationship exists between the two and the SVR is the reciprocal of the slope. A small volume of the radioisotope technetium-99m, together with a vasodilator such as histamine, is injected into the skin and the rate of clearance of the isotope is recorded. The pressure from a sphygmomanometer cuff just necessary to prevent the radioisotope from leaving the area is taken as the SPP. This value reflects the degree of large artery disease. A value of 30 mmHg or more is needed to ensure healing. Radionuclide imaging as performed for investigation of coronary arteries can also be used to estimate blood flow in the foot and to detect the presence of osteomyelitis (Faris 1991).

**Laser–Doppler fluximetry.** This measures the movement of red blood cells in cutaneous vessels, which changes as ischaemia progresses and so can be used to determine amputation level.

# VENOUS DRAINAGE

Venous problems may arise in the superficial, communicating and/or deep veins (Table 6.7). Superficial veins lie in the superficial fascia, deep veins lie in skeletal muscle and communicating veins link the two. There are three main pathological processes affecting veins, which can be interlinked:

- absent or incompetent valves
- formation of a thrombus which may trigger secondary inflammation of the vein wall (thrombophlebitis)
- inflammation of the vein wall (phlebitis) with possible secondary formation of a thrombus (phlebo-thrombosis).

The first condition affects superficial or communicating veins. The cause may be congenital, where family history is common; be caused by increased pressure, such as occurs during pregnancy; or an abdominal tumour or ascites which causes venodilation and renders the valves incompetent. Much less common are congenital conditions causing swelling or dilation of veins. The resulting back flow due to gravity leads to increased hydrostatic pressure in the lower limb veins, giving rise to the knotty appearance of varicose veins.

The second and third conditions can affect superficial or deep veins, but part of the sequelae of deep vein pathology is often superficial varicosities. Phlebitis with no thrombosis affects superficial veins, usually as a result of trauma or infection. Causes of venous thrombi are multifactorial, being any factors which contribute to Virchow's triad of:

- stasis
- hypercoagulability
- injury to the endothelium.

Patients suffering from recurrent thromboses show a familial tendency and an association has been demonstrated with a mutation for genes

**Table 6.7** Causes of venous insufficiency

| Type | Cause |
|---|---|
| Superfical | Varicose veins:<br>  primary – idiopathic<br>  secondary – backflow from deep to<br>  superficial vein |
| | Thrombophlebitis |
| | Phlebangioma (congenital swelling of vein)<br>Phlebectasia (congenital dilation of vein) |
| Deep | Deep vein thrombosis due to:<br>  abnormalities affecting blood flow<br>  abnormalities of clotting<br>  abnormalities of endothelium |
| | Idiopathic |
| | Thrombophlebitis |

## Lymphangitis and lymphadenitis

As the majority of tissue fluid normally drains into the lymphatic system, it follows that any infection present in the tissues, as indicated by the presence of cellulitis, will also drain into the lymph vessels unless dealt with by the inflammatory response at the site of infection. The presence of infection in the lymphatic vessels causes local inflammation, seen as red streaks following the course of the vessel; it is called lymphangitis. Should the infection reach the lymph nodes/glands into which the lymph vessels drain, they will become tender and swollen (lymphadenitis). If not overcome by the body's natural defences or by appropriate antibiosis, the infection will enter the bloodstream (bacteraemia) and finally cause widespread systemic infection (septicaemia/blood poisoning).

## Yellow nail syndrome

The nail appears yellow in colour, thickened but smooth and there is an increase in lateral curvature. The rate of growth of the nail is reduced. The condition is associated with chronic lymphoedema.

## Clinical tests

It is not usual to carry out any clinical tests for lymphoedema apart from those which will distinguish it from other types of oedema, such as whether it is pitting or non-pitting.

## Hospital tests

Angiography for lymphatic vessels (lymphangiography) can be carried out in the same manner as for venography. In primary lymphoedema X-rays may show hypoplasia of the lymphatic system, with the lymphatic channels appearing scanty and spidery.

## SUMMARY

This chapter has outlined an assessment process from which practitioners can arrive at a diagnosis of the vascular status of a patient. Case studies have been included to illustrate the effects of vascular problems.

The information gained from the vascular assessment can be used to make a diagnosis and draw up an effective treatment plan. While many different pathologies can affect the cardiovascular system, there are five important signs which should always alert the practitioner to further investigation:

- absence of pedal pulses
- ABPI <0.9
- intermittent claudication
- oedema
- a difference in temperature between the two lower limbs of 2°C or more.

It is important to establish if tissue perfusion falls within an acceptable range in relation to the patient's age. If it does, as long as no other problems exist, the patient can receive the same treatment as for any other non-risk patient. If vascular problems are present or there is a distinct possibility they will occur in the future, then it is important to give prophylactic advice and treatment. Choice of treatment, e.g. surgery, will be affected by the presence of vascular problems, as wound healing will be impaired and the patient is at greater risk of developing infections.

### REFERENCES

Ameli F M, Stein M, Provan J L, Aro L, Prosser R, St Louis E L 1989 Comparison between transcutaneous oximetry and ankle–brachial pressure ratio in predicting run off and outcome in patients who undergo aortofemoral bypass. Canadian Journal of Surgery 32: 428–432

Banga J D 1995 Lower extremity arterial disease in diabetes mellitus. Journal of British Podiatric Medicine 50: 68–72

Blackwell S 2001 Common anemias – What lies behind? Clinical Reviews 11: 53–62

Coull A 1988 Making sense of pulse oximetry. Nursing Times 32: 42–43

Davies C S 1992 A comparative investigation of ankle–brachial pressure indices within an age variable population. British Journal of Podiatric Medicine 48: 21–24

Davies A H, Horrocks M 1992 Vascular assessment and the ischaemic foot. Foot 2: 1–6

Faris I 1991 The management of the diabetic foot, 2nd edn. Churchill Livingstone, Edinburgh, p 150

Ganong W F 1991 Review of medical physiology, 15th edn. Lange, London, p 510

Hecht H S, Superko H R 2001 Electron beam tomography (EBT) may improve diagnosis of subclinical CAD in females. Journal of the American College of Cardiology 37: 1506–1511

Howell M A, Colgan M P, Seeger R W, Ramsay D E, Sumner D S 1989 Relationship of severity of lower limb peripheral vascular disease to mortality and morbidity: a six year follow-up study. Journal of Vascular Surgery 9: 691–696, discussion 697

Huntleigh Diagnostics 1999 Library of sounds-support booklet for audio cassette. Huntleigh Diagnostics, Cardiff, pp 5–21

Insall R L, Davies R J, Prout W G 1989 Significance of the Buerger's test in the assessment of lower limb ischaemia. Journal of the Royal Society of Medicine 82: 729–731

Kapoor A S, Singh B N 1993a Prognosis and risk assessment in cardiovascular disease. Churchill Livingstone, New York, p 131

Kapoor A S, Singh B N 1993b Prognosis and risk assessment in cardiovascular disease. Churchill Livingstone, New York, pp 130–131, 145

Kapoor A S, Singh B N 1993c Prognosis and risk assessment in cardiovascular disease. Churchill Livingstone, New York, pp 4, 11, 423

Khachemoune A, Sahu M, Phillips T J 2001 Diagnostic dilemmas. Wounds 13: 2–4

Kumar P J, Clark M L 1990a Clinical medicine. A textbook for medical students and doctors, 2nd edn. Baillière Tindall, London, p 571

Kumar P J, Clark M L 1990b Clinical medicine. A textbook for medical students and doctors, 2nd edn. Baillière Tindall, London, p 516

Kumar P J, Clark M L 1990c Clinical medicine. A textbook for medical students and doctors, 2nd edn. Baillière Tindall, London, pp 539–540

Kumar P J, Clark M L 1990d Clinical medicine. A textbook for medical students and doctors, 2nd edn. Baillière Tindall, London, p 538

Lainge S P, Greenhalgh R M 1980 Standard exercise test to assess peripheral arterial disease. British Medical Journal 280: 13–16

Lowe G D O (ed) 1993 Critical limb ischaemia – a slide lecture kit. Schering Health Care/Professional Postgraduate Services Europe Ltd, Worthing

Mercer K G , Berridge D C 2000 Peripheral vascular disease and vascular reconstruction. In: Boulton A J M, Connor H, Cavannagh P R (eds) The foot in diabetes, 3rd edn. J Wiley, Chichester, p 220

Murphie P 2001a Macrovasular disease aetiology and diabetic foot ulceration. Journal of Wound Care 10: 103–107

Murphie P 2001b Microvascular disease aetiology in diabetic foot ulceration. Journal of Wound Care 10: 159–162

Nicholson M J, Byrne R L, Steele G A, Callum K G 1993 Predictive value of bruits and Doppler pressure measurements in detecting lower limb arterial stenosis. European Journal of Vascular Surgery 7: 59–62

Smith F C T, Shearman C P, Simms M H, Gwynn B R 1994 Falsely elevated ankle pressures in severe leg ischaemia: the pole test – an alternative approach. European Journal of Vascular Surgery 8: 408–412

---

## FURTHER READING

Berkow R (ed) 2000 The Merck manual. Merck, Sharp and Dohme Research Laboratories, New Jersey

Berne R M, Levy M N 1992 Cardiovascular physiology, 6th edn. Mosby Year Book, St Louis, MO

Vander A, Sherman J, Luciano D 2000 Human physiology – the mechanisms of body function, international edition, 8th edn. McGraw-Hill, Boston

Walker W E 1991 A colour atlas of peripheral vascular disease. Wolfe Medical, London

Yao S T 1970 Haemodynamic studies in peripheral arterial disease. British Journal of Surgery 57: 761–766

# 7

# Neurological assessment

*J. McLeod Roberts*

There are many conditions affecting the nervous system which modify lower limb function (Table 7.1). The purpose of this chapter is to enable the practitioner to detect the presence of these conditions. The chapter begins with an outline of the histology, organisation and function of the nervous system. Reflexes are dealt with as a separate topic as they form the basis of so much neurological behaviour. It is not possible to discuss the nervous system without also making some reference to the muscular system: since muscles are the effector organs for much nervous activity, neurological deficits are often recognised by their characteristic effects on muscle. Similarly, muscular disease may show similar characteristics to those of nervous disorders. The second part of this chapter is concerned with a detailed description of the assessment of each part of the neuromuscular system and, for the purposes of this chapter, the descriptive term 'neurological' is also taken to imply 'neuromuscular' wherever appropriate.

## Why undertake an assessment of the patient's neurological status?

It is important to undertake an assessment of the neurological status in order to identify whether the patient has an intact and normally functioning neurological system. The purpose of the assessment is to:

- establish which, if any, part of the nervous system is functioning abnormally

**Table 7.1** Neurological conditions that may affect the lower limb

| Condition | Description |
| --- | --- |
| Cerebral vascular accident (CVA) (stroke) | Due to haemorrhage, embolus or thrombosis of the cerebral arteries |
| Parkinsonism | Degeneration of dopaminergic receptors. Usually idiopathic but can be drug induced |
| Friedreich's ataxia | One of a group of hereditary syndromes affecting the cerebellum. Inheritance is autosomal recessive. Onset in childhood, death usual around 40 years |
| Multiple sclerosis | Patchy demyelination of the CNS. Shows relapses and remissions. Onset 20+ |
| Poliomyelitis | Virus that affects lower motor neurones (LMNs). |
| Syringomyelia | Progressive destruction of the spinal cord due to blockage of central canal, e.g. tumour |
| Tabes dorsal | Occurs with tertiary stage syphilis |
| Spina bifida | Defective closure of vertebral column. Congenital |
| Motor neurone disease | Degeneration of both upper motor neurones (UMNs) and LMNs. No sensory loss. Onset usually between 40 and 60 years. Death usually due to respiratory infection. Idiopathic |
| Subacute combined degeneration of the spinal cord | Due to lack of vitamin $B_{12}$. Usually seen in pernicious anaemia. Affects both sensory and motor tracts in the spinal cord. See UMN signs, sensory and proprioceptive deficit. Reversible if detected in time |
| Charcot–Marie–Tooth disease/ peroneal muscle atrophy/hereditary motor–sensory neuropathy | Affects peroneal nerve, predominantly motor with variable sensory deficit. Commonest inherited neuropathy. Usually autosomal dominant. Onset in teens, slowly worsens |
| Guillain–Barré syndrome | Post-viral autoimmune response, rapid onset, potentially fatal from respiratory failure. Predominantly motor effects, with muscle weakness and paralysis, but some sensory loss; 80% of patients show full recovery. Also chronic relapsing form |
| Neurofibromatosis | Autosomal dominant condition that leads to tumours of nerves and compression of spinal cord |
| Peripheral neuropathy | Occurs due to a variety of causes, e.g. alcoholism, injury, diabetes mellitus |
| Myasthenia gravis | Autoimmune disease that affects the neuromuscular junction and leads to severe fatigue and weakness/paralysis |
| Myopathies | Range of relatively rare diseases affecting muscle only. May be inherited or acquired. Symptoms similar to LMN diseases but no fasciculation |

- identify the extent of dysfunction
- where possible, arrive at a specific diagnosis
- draw up a treatment plan which takes account of the above information.

It is important to establish which part or parts of the nervous system are affected. For example, an ataxic (uncoordinated) gait may be due to a disorder of the cerebellum or a lack of proprioceptive information. The practitioner may be in a position to identify early changes in neurological function, e.g. initial clinical features associated with multiple sclerosis such as double vision, falling over, tingling sensations, and loss of function. If an appropriate treatment plan is to be drawn up, knowledge of the presence of any condition and its specific effects on the lower limb is essential. For example, sufferers of Guillain–Barré syndrome are predisposed to foot ulcers and so the treatment plan should include preventative measures and a monitoring programme, as 10% of patients may show incomplete recovery.

ness on either the contralateral side, if the site of damage is before the tracts cross, or the ipsilateral (same) side, if the site of damage occurs after the tracts have crossed.

## Motor pathways

Just as all conscious stimuli are interpreted in the cortex, so all conscious actions originate there. The whole area is known as the sensorimotor cortex; one part is called the primary motor cortex and initiates conscious action (Fig. 7.12). It too shows somatotopic organisation, so that damage to this region produces precise effects on particular actions on the contralateral side of the body. Close to this area is the premotor cortex, which is involved in the planning of actions. Since the actions produced by these neurones are the conscious movements of the body, the muscles involved will be skeletal and the neurones will be part of the somatic motor system.

Neurones in the brain which are responsible for initiating the commands are called upper motor neurones (UMNs). They do not send impulses directly to the muscles but exert their influence via neurones in the ventral (anterior) horn of the spinal cord called lower motor neurones (LMNs). The latter send impulses to the skeletal muscles via their axons, which form the peripheral efferent pathways within spinal nerves.

The descending pathways from brain to spinal cord can be divided into two main tracts: the corticospinal tract and the multineuronal (brain stem) tract (see Fig. 7.11).

**The corticospinal tract.** This is a rapid pathway and is mainly responsible for the skilled movements of small, distal limb muscles such as those used in scalpel work. Most of the fibres cross over in the brain stem and descend in the white matter of the spinal cord as the lateral corticospinal tract. The uncrossed fibres descend as the ventral (anterior) corticospinal tract. At the appropriate level in the spinal cord they enter the ventral horn of the grey matter to synapse with a lower motor neurone. Because the corticospinal tract forms a rough pyramid shape as it passes through the brain stem, it is also called the pyramidal tract.

**The multineuronal tract.** This tract runs to lower motor neurones by a slower, more diffuse route, since it makes many more synaptic connections on the way, particularly in the descending reticular system and the nuclei of the brain stem. Although influenced by UMNs the tracts are only recognisable as separate pathways as they emerge from the brain stem to travel through the spinal cord as the vestibulospinal, tectospinal and reticulospinal tracts. The tracts enter the ventral horn of the grey matter to influence the appropriate lower motor neurone.

These tracts do not form part of the pyramids in the medulla and so are also called the extra- (outside) pyramidal pathways. They mainly influence the large, proximal limb muscles and the axial muscles of posture, and have a predominately inhibitory effect on the ventral horn cells. They are responsible for the antigravity reflexes, which keep our knees extended and head erect in order to maintain upright posture.

The division of the descending tracts is not clear cut, as they also demonstrate redundancy, there being much overlap and interaction between the two. Other areas of the brain also have strong modifying influences, such as the cerebellum and clusters of neurones in the fore- and midbrain known collectively as the basal ganglia.

The last stage in the production of a conscious action is the excitation of an LMN in the ventral (anterior) horn of the spinal cord and the passage of an impulse along its axon in the spinal nerve to the skeletal muscle. The LMN will be subject to influences from many neurones, not only from descending tracts but also from spinal neurones. As many as 10 000–15 000 synapses, both excitatory and inhibitory, can occur on one lower motor neurone. If the sum of these influences is excitatory, the LMN will be stimulated to discharge an impulse along its axon and the skeletal muscle will contract. This peripheral pathway from LMN to skeletal muscle is called the final common pathway and the entire pathway, including the neuromuscular junction and the 10–600 skeletal muscle fibres innervated by that nerve is called a motor unit (Fig. 7.13).

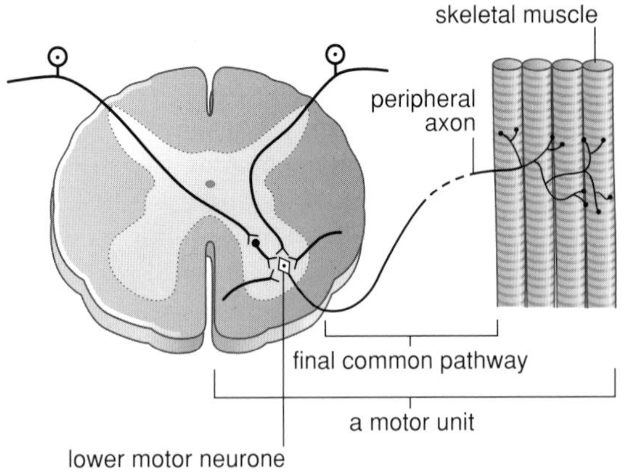

**Figure 7.13** The final common pathway of a motor unit.

## Cerebellum

The actions of the cerebellum are unconscious and are very important in postural reflexes. The cerebellum has no direct descending pathways to the spinal cord; instead it has a rich afferent input and sends modifying influences to the sensorimotor cortex, the reticular formation and the brain-stem nuclei. Thus, symptoms of cerebellar defects may be due to lesions in the ascending spinocerebellar tracts, in the cerebellum itself or in efferent pathways going to other parts of the brain.

The cerebellum receives all information about position sense. The vestibular apparatus of the ear projects via the vestibular nuclei of the brain stem to the flocculonodular lobe. The spinocerebellar tracts carry proprioceptive information from muscles, tendons, joints and cutaneous pressure receptors which project to the vermis and anterior lobes. The cerebral cortex gives information about the actions decided upon and projects to the posterior lobes via pontine nuclei. The cerebellum integrates the information received from all these areas and compares it with the information on intended actions received from the cerebral cortex. It then sends modifying influences back to the motor cortex and brain stem, so that descending instructions to the LMNs can be altered where necessary.

## Basal ganglia

At present the precise functions of the basal ganglia in movement are unknown, but they are thought to enable abstract thought (ideas) to be converted into voluntary action (Ganong 1991a). Like the cerebellum they function at an unconscious level and have no direct pathway to LMNs but influence the sensorimotor cortex and the descending reticular formation. Because the main action of the basal ganglia is on the descending extrapyramidal tracts, they have become known as the extrapyramidal system and conditions affecting them are referred to as extrapyramidal syndromes, e.g. parkinsonism.

## REFLEXES

Reflex actions are automatic responses to particular stimuli and form the basis of much of our behaviour, from the simple knee jerk to driving a car. They are also very important in posture, balance and gait. Reflexes can be inborn (inherited, innate, instinctive) or acquired (learned). Examples of the former are eye blink, pupil dilation/constriction, change in heart rate, knee jerk (stretch) reflex, pain withdrawal and sweat secretion. Examples of the latter are swimming, walking, driving, debriding callus. They can involve any subdivisions of the nervous system and any type of effector organ. We may be aware of them or they may never reach consciousness. It is here that the close association between the nervous and endocrine systems is best illustrated, since both can contribute to the same reflex arc. For example, when the retina of the eye detects a threatening situation, this information will be carried by the optic nerve to the brain and one of the responses will be the release of the hormone adrenaline (epinephrine) from the adrenal medulla, to prepare the body for action.

In all cases, the pathway allows the body to respond rapidly to a given stimulus. Generally, inborn reflexes produce stereotypic responses which are usually protective reflexes or those needed for posture and balance. Acquired reflexes are more complex, involving the conscious cortex and many different effectors, so that the response (see Fig. 7.12). Any damage to this area, whatever the cause, will produce a contralateral sensory deficit in the appropriate part of the body. Damage to the occipital lobe (striate cortex) will produce visual disturbances. The most common cause of such neurological deficits is an occlusion or haemorrhage of one of the cerebral arteries.

Damage to the ascending tracts in the spinal cord will produce either ipsi- or contralateral effects, depending on the site of the lesion in relation to the point of crossover of the tracts. This is well illustrated in the Brown–Séquard syndrome, where damage to one side of the spinal cord results in:

- ipsilateral loss of touch, position sense, two-point discrimination and vibration sense below the level of the lesion, due to dorsal column injury
- contralateral loss of pain and temperature sensation below the level of the lesion, due to damage to the anterolateral tracts.

The exact effect of peripheral nerve damage depends on the site and the nature of the damage, since this dictates the repair process (Table 7.12).

## History

The nature and distribution of any sensory deficit can be an important aid in diagnosing the underlying cause. This may take the form of

**Table 7.12**  Classification of nerve damage

| Type | Damage |
|------|--------|
| Neuropraxia | Mild trauma or compression causing local demyelination and leading to temporary loss of function. Full recovery within days or weeks |
| Axonotmesis | Crush injuries causing degeneration of axon and myelin sheath (wallerian degeneration) Neurolemma sheaths intact and reinnervated |
| Neurotmesis | Whole nerve axon severed. Surgical repair needed to ensure reinnervation of distal trunk |

complete anaesthesia (total lack of sensation) or paraesthesia (an altered sensation). Examples of paraesthesia are pins and needles, burning, pricking, shooting pain and dull ache. Patients should be asked if they experience any abnormal sensations.

**Phantom limb.**  An unusual phenomenon that arises from amputation of a limb is that of 'phantom limb', where the patient has the very real sensation of the amputated limb still being present and behaving just like a normal limb. The most unpleasant effect is the sensation of pain which is said to occur in 70% of amputees (Melzack 1992). The traditional explanation, that this is due to the growth of neuromas in the nerve stumps which continue to generate impulses, cannot be the entire explanation since cutting the afferent pathways from such nerves does not abolish the pain. Melzack has suggested that the phantom sensations are due to learned circuits in the brain that are capable of generating impulses in the absence of sensory inputs.

**Referred pain.**  Injury to the viscera often produces pain in a somatic structure some distance away. This is called referred pain. For example, a myocardial infarction can produce pain in the left arm as both the heart and the skin of the left arm have developed from the same dermatomal segment. However, the exact mechanism is still not clearly understood although both convergence and facilitation are thought to play a role (Ganong 1991b). Damage to a spinal nerve may result in referred pain which is experienced around the heel; this occurs if there is damage to S1.

## Clinical tests

Simple apparatus is all that is needed to undertake an assessment of sensory function. Among the apparatus that can be used are cotton wool, the fine brush of a neurological hammer, a pair of blunted dividers or a pair of blunt-ended orange sticks, a 128 Hz tuning fork, a 10g monofilament, a neurothesiometer, Neurotips (Owen Mumford) and two small metal test tubes, metal being a better conductor of heat than glass. Although all the methods are acceptable, only tests using

**Table 7.13**  Sensory testing

| Sense | Method | Fibre type and pathway in spinal cord |
| --- | --- | --- |
| Light touch | Cottonwool/brush/monofilament | A-beta fibres |
| Two-point discrimination | Dividers, two orange sticks | Ipsilateral dorsal column |
| Vibration (pressure) | Tuning fork/neurothesiometer | |
| Temperature | Warm and cold test tubes/ dissimilar metals | A-delta and C fibres Contralateral (anterolateral columns) |
| Sharp pain/pinprick | Neurotips | |
| Proprioception | Dorsi/plantarflexion of hallux | A-alpha fibres Ipsilateral dorsal columns |

monofilaments and neurothesiometers/biothesiometers have been evaluated. The tests examine the integrity of the afferent pathways that involve the ipsilateral dorsal columns and the contralateral anterolateral columns (Table 7.13). Each test should be demonstrated to the patient first, usually on the back of the patient's hand, so that the test is understood and the expected sensation experienced. It is then possible to ask the patient to compare the same sensations on hand and foot which will indicate the degree, if any, of sensory loss. If the patient suffers from neuropathy of the upper limbs, the demonstration test can take place on the forehead. For the actual test, where appropriate, the patients should have their eyes closed in order that the results cannot be influenced by observing the test. Use of forced-answer questions where possible help to eliminate observer influence, e.g. 'Which is sharper, number 1 or number 2?'.

Sham testing, where appropriate, should also be used to rule out any attempts to guess the correct answer by the patient. The test should be repeated three times on the same site and if 2/3 answers are correct, the patient is not considered to have a sensory deficit in that modality. If screening is being carried out to detect generalised neuropathy it is important that the tests involve all the dermatomes at that level (see Fig. 7.8), starting distally and working proximally. As most peripheral neuropathies begin at the most distal site and progress proximally, it is only necessary to test more proximal areas if the test has proved negative distally. The results of each test

should state the extent of any neuropathy, e.g. 'loss of vibration perception from toes to ankles' to aid monitoring of the deficit. If a mononeuropathy is suspected, e.g. anterior tibial damage contributing to foot drop, the dermatomes innervated by that nerve should be investigated. A deficit may not always be due to pathological causes: factors such as overlying callus render the skin less sensitive and the normal slowing of conduction rates associated with ageing results in a reduction in sensation.

### Testing large-diameter fibres

**Light touch.** Cotton wool, a fine brush or a 10$g$ monofilament can all be used for this test. The nerves being tested are large-diameter A-beta fibres which ascend in the dorsal columns, transmitting light touch perception. The receptors (Meissner's corpuscles) lie in the superficial dermis. After explaining the test, the patient's eyes should be shut. The patient is asked to state when the foot is being stroked and to indicate the site. The clinician should make no further comment until the test is finished. The skin of the foot is then stroked lightly with a wisp of cotton wool/brush or monofilament. The sense of touch will be reduced in the elderly and in calloused skin (due to thickened skin). The patient may incorrectly distinguish between the lesser toes in this test, but this is normal and is due to the particular innervation of the lesser digits.

**Two-point discrimination.** Blunt-ended orange sticks or the two points of a pair of dividers can be used for this test, providing the points of the dividers have been blunted to avoid accidental skin penetration. The nerves being tested are again the large-diameter A-beta fibres, but here the density of the touch receptor field is being assessed. The plantar surface of the foot is usually tested. The patient is asked, with eyes shut, to state how many points can be felt when the tips of a compass lightly press the skin surface simultaneously. The distance between the tips of the compass that allows the patient to detect two points rather than one should be noted. Usually the distance on the foot of a healthy young adult is 2 cm. It will increase with age and if the skin is calloused. The receptors responsible for identifying two-point discrimination are also essential for stereognosis – the ability to recognise objects by touch – and are therefore very important for readers of Braille.

**Pressure.** The 10$g$ monofilament is used for this test. The first monofilament for detecting neuropathy was the Semmes–Weinstein monofilament produced by the Hansen's Disease Center, USA. In theory this monofilament buckles when a force of 10$g$ is applied. Since then a wide variety of monofilaments have been produced, all said to be buckled by the same force of 10$g$. However, McGill et al (1998) and Booth & Young (2000) studied 10$g$ monofilaments from a range of manufacturers and found inconsistencies in their deforming pressures. The clinical relevance of this variation has yet to be determined. Booth & Young (2000) also showed that all monofilaments decline with use and recommended a 24-hour rest should be allowed between repeated use of a single monofilament to allow recovery. A range of monofilaments of different diameters and buckling forces is also available, but these are more useful for research purposes than for routine screening. In view of its small size, low cost and ability in detecting large-fibre neuropathy, the monofilament is considered one of the most useful tools a clinician can possess and is recommended by the International Diabetes Federation, the World Health Organization European St. Vincent Declaration and the International Working Group on the diabetic foot (International Consensus on the Diabetic Foot 1999).

The nerve fibres being tested are once more those belonging to the A-beta group of fibres. The receptors are encapsulated and lie in the dermis but are slow adaptors and so detect constant pressure rather than vibration. Both touch and pressure receptors can respond to applied pressure, the difference being in the force used to apply the pressure. Light touch will stimulate a small area of nerve endings and increasing pressure will recruit more and more receptors. When the stimulus becomes pressure rather than touch and whether a different receptor is involved with increased pressure is not clear, so the stimulus is sometimes referred to as the touch-pressure sensation.

The monofilament is applied at right angles to the skin surface with just enough pressure to deform the filament into a 'C' shape. Care should be taken not to slide the filament or brush the skin. It should be held in that position for 2 seconds, the patient having been asked to state when and where pressure from the 10$g$ monofilament is felt at various points, with eyes shut. Inability to detect the 10$g$ monofilament is taken to indicate neuropathy of large fibres.

**Vibration.** Either a simple 128 Hz tuning fork or a graduated Rydel–Seiffer version can be used. The nerve fibres being tested are again large-diameter A-beta fibres, sensitive to pressure, but this time the deeply placed pacinian corpuscles are particularly sensitive to rapidly changing pressures or vibrations. They are coated with layers of connective tissue, which has the ability to absorb low-frequency pressure changes, so that only high-frequency vibrations such as those produced by the tuning fork will reach the central receptor.

The vibrating tuning fork is placed on the skin above a bony prominence such as the apex of the hallux, malleolus or the first metatarsophalangeal joint (MTPJ). It is important to ask the patients to describe what they feel, without any prompting, as most patients will be able to feel pressure, but not necessarily any vibratory sensation. Most patients describe the vibratory sensation as a 'buzzing'. The argument that the tuning fork should not be placed over bone, as this augments the sensation, is immaterial, since all damaging pressures to which the foot is likely to be subjected – e.g. tight footwear, ground forces on bony deformities or foreign objects in footwear – compress soft tissue against bone. The Rydel–Seiffer tuning fork is an attempt to produce a semi-quantitative result to enable comparisons to be made with other patients and on different occasions. It has detachable clamps which can be moved to different positions on the prongs, to alter the vibrating frequency from 64 to 128 Hz. As the prongs vibrate, the apex of a cone drawn on the clamps, upright or inverted, will appear to move vertically up or down a scale from 1 to 8. The position of this cone is noted when the patients say the vibration sensation stops. At 128 Hz the apex should reach at least halfway along the scale, i.e. to the number 4 from 1 or 8, depending on which cone is being observed. If vibration sensation is lost before this point is reached, the patient is said to have a vibratory perception deficit.

Neurothesiometers provide an alternative method of assessing vibration. The neurothesiometer is basically a vibrator that delivers vibrations of increasing strength, measured in volts per micrometre. The mains-operated version, the biothesiometer, has been superseded by the battery-operated neurothesiometer, to meet Health and Safety requirements. Cassella et al (2000) recommended that rather than using a pistol grip when using the apparatus, the head of the tool should rest in the palm of the operator's hand while being applied to the patient. Only in this way, with no extraneous pressure being applied, could truly reproducible vibratory perception thresholds (VPTs) be determined. The neurothesiometer is positioned over a bony prominence and the strength of the vibrations is increased until the patient can detect a 'buzzing' sensation. This reading is called the VPT and values of over 25 volts are taken to indicate the presence of peripheral neuropathy. The measurement should be repeated three times and the average value taken. An alternative method is to begin with the maximum intensity of stimulus and reduce it until the patient

can no longer detect any sensation. This method is not measuring the same index, however, and the two methods should not be mixed on the same patient. Up to 12 readings can be stored in the memory of the apparatus. Intra-observer error is small. The disadvantages of the apparatus are its cost and weight. Using data from 392 patients with diabetes mellitus, Coppini et al (2000) found that using a VPT score based on comparing the patient's value of VPT with an age-related normal population showed overall better sensitivity and specificity than raw VPT in identifying patients with subclinical neuropathy; they felt that this measurement would be more useful in regular monitoring of diabetic patients. A VPT score >10.1 indicates increased risk of developing neuropathy.

### Testing small-diameter fibres

**Temperature.** Two test tubes filled with warm and cool water are preferable to immersing saline sachets in cool and warm water, which quickly lose their temperature differences. Metal rods cooled or warmed in water can also be used. A small cylinder made of two metals with dissimilar conductivities is even easier to transport and use, but is not so readily available in the UK. For research purposes, quantitative instruments to measure temperature perception thresholds using thermode devices (Kalter-Leibovici et al 2001) or thermo-aesthesiometers (van Schie et al 1998) have been used. The latter paper concludes that a combined method, using two simple clinical tests and the more sophisticated apparatus, produced the highest sensitivity (76%).

This tests the integrity of the warmth and cold temperature receptors that feed into the anterior part of the anterolateral columns. The nerve fibres involved are narrow diameter A-delta and C fibres. Cutaneous receptors detect absolute values rather than the temperature gradient across the skin. Warmth receptors operate in the range of 30–43°C and cold receptors operate in the range of 35–20°C (Vander et al 1998). Temperatures above 43°C or below 20°C will trigger pain receptors. The skin temperature is usually a few degrees cooler than that of core temperature, i.e.

between 30 and 35°C, though a greater difference may exist in extremes of environmental temperatures. The temperature of the warm water should be above 35°C and that of the cold water below 30°C. Again, with eyes closed, the patient is asked to state which they find the cooler/warmer from the first or second tube presented.

**Pain.** Disposable Neurotips (Owen Mumford) are best used for this test. The Neurotips have a sharp and a blunt end, but the sharp end cannot pierce the skin. Spring-loaded devices which are designed to deliver a stimulus at a force of 40g are thought to be the safest and most reliable way of testing for pinprick sensitivity (Wareham et al 1997). The use of the sharp end of a patella hammer is not advisable as it may be sharp enough to penetrate the skin and is non-disposable. A hypodermic syringe should not be used as the danger of skin penetration is high.

This tests the integrity of the sharp pain pathway, which begins with free nerve endings in the dermis. A-delta fibres travel into the spinal cord and synapse in the dorsal horn. The postsynaptic fibres then cross to the contralateral anterolateral columns which travel up to the brain.

Using disposable Neurotips and with eyes closed the patient is asked to state which is sharper, the first or second sensation. The two ends should be presented in random sequence to avoid correct guessing by the anxious-to-please patient. Neuropathy does not always mean absence of pain, as is witnessed by diabetic patients with neuropathy who can experience a period of intense pain (Boulton 2000).

There are certain perceived wisdoms concerning sensory testing on diabetic patients which the busy practitioner may use to justify using only one of the above methods:

- vibration sensation is the first modality to deteriorate
- the presence of neuropathy as indicated by failure to detect the 10g monofilament implies neuropathy of all nerve fibres in that limb.

There is no conclusive evidence to support either of these statements. Indeed Winkler et al (2000) have reported the existence of a subgroup of type 1 diabetic neuropathy patients who suffer from autonomic symptoms severe enough to warrant treatment, such as severe bladder or gastroparesis, orthostatic hypotension and diabetic diarrhoea associated with a selective small-fibre sensory and autonomic loss with relatively preserved large-fibre sensory modalities such as vibration and touch-pressure sensation. Whether either or both of the above statements can be applied to patients without diabetes is even less certain. A study by Nakayama et al (1998) on rats showed that small-diameter, unmyelinated nerve fibres decrease in number with ageing whereas larger-diameter fibres maintain both conduction ability and numbers. In the absence of solid evidence to the contrary, it would seem advisable to carry out sensory testing on both small and large fibres. However, any testing is better than none. In research studies, a range of sensory tests have been used to calculate a neuropathy disability score (NDS). For further discussion of peripheral neuropathy assessment in patients with diabetes mellitus see Boulton et al 1998, Young & Matthews 1998 and Chapter 17.

**Tinel's sign.** This helps in the diagnosis of nerve compression. Palpating the nerve, or tapping it with a patellar hammer, at the site of compression will often elicit an abnormal sensation distally, but it can also follow the proximal distribution of the nerve. Usually the sensation is paraesthesia (tingling, burning) or is like an electric shock. Tinel's sign can be used to assess for compression of the medial nerve at the wrist or the posterior tibial nerve at the ankle (carpal and tarsal tunnel syndromes). However, no clinical tests for carpal and tarsal tunnel syndromes are entirely reliable (Golding et al 1986), so that the suspicion of such a condition needs to be confirmed by nerve conduction tests (see Hospital tests).

**Referred pain.** Entrapment of a spinal nerve may lead to paraesthesia, pain and weakness of muscles in the lower limb. Normally when pressure is applied to a site of pain, the pain becomes worse. However, with referred pain the level of pain stays about the same. A suspected entrapment of the sciatic nerve usually leads to pain when the affected leg is raised while the patient lies in a supine position.

## Hospital tests

**Nerve conduction test.** Sensory nerve conduction velocities are measured by placing stimulating electrodes on the skin over the nerve to be tested. Recording electrodes, either skin or needle electrodes, are placed either proximally for orthodromic stimulation or distally for antidromic stimulation. The latter gives more consistent results. The lower limit of normal sensory conduction velocities in the lower limb is around 35 m/s. Values are less than those for the upper limb. A slowing of conduction velocity may be due to a variety of causes (Matthews & Arnold 1991):

- ageing
- damage to the cell body as in herpes zoster (shingles)
- nerve axon damage as in compression due to a spinal tumour, a slipped disc or tarsal/carpal tunnel syndrome
- demyelinisation as seen in Guillain–Barré syndrome.

Amplitude of the action potentials and latency are also measured. For a brief discussion of possible findings, see section on motor nerve conduction tests.

**Nerve biopsy.** This can be carried out on sensory, motor and autonomic nerves. A small sample of tissue is removed, using a needle, cone or, if surgery is being performed, a scalpel. The tissue is examined histologically and its interpretation requires great expertise. Characteristics such as a thickened basement membrane, scarring of the myelin sheath, etc., can be identified. Biopsies are carried out where another laboratory test is inconclusive or where no other diagnostic test exists for the suspected condition.

## ASSESSMENT OF LOWER LIMB MOTOR FUNCTION

If the motor system is functioning normally muscles should display a resting tone, show good muscle power on active contraction and be able to move against resistance (Ch. 8).

The lower limb reflexes, patella and Achilles, should also show a normal response. Reflex pathways involve both an afferent and an efferent component and therefore a deficit in either component would be expected to have an observable effect on the response, as would abnormal influences by higher centres on the LMN. Reflex responses can be graded as follows (Fuller 1993a):

3+ = clonus
2+ = increased
1+ = normal
+/− = obtainable with reinforcement
0 = absent.

Values of 2 and above suggest UMN lesions, values of below 1 suggest LMN lesions, peripheral sensory nerve or muscle damage.

**The patellar reflex.** This tests the integrity of the spinal reflex pathway (L3, L4) and demonstrates descending influences on the ventral horn cell. It is important that the limb being tested is as relaxed as possible. The patient should sit sideways on the examination couch with the feet clearing the ground. The practitioner can gently push the leg to be tested, which should swing freely in response. A gentle tap on the patellar tendon with the hammer should elicit a knee jerk. If the leg is not relaxed, the patient should clasp both hands around the other knee and pull (Jedrassik manoeuvre). This releases spinal influence and allows the leg to relax. The test should be undertaken on both legs.

**The Achilles reflex.** This tests the spinal reflex pathway (S1, S2). The response is best elicited if the foot of the patient is slightly dorsiflexed by applying gentle pressure to the plantar surface of the forefoot with one hand and tapping the Achilles tendon while the pressure is maintained. The patient can either sit on a couch, with legs extended and the limb being tested crossed over the other, or kneel on a chair, with the foot to be tested hanging slightly over the edge of the chair. In a healthy young adult the forefoot will gently plantarflex. In an elderly person no visible movement may be seen, but a very slight plantarflexion will be felt against the practitioner's hand.

Lower limb motor dysfunction can occur as a result of damage to upper motor neurones, lower motor neurones, peripheral nerves or muscles.

# Upper motor neurone lesions

Upper motor neurone (UMN) lesions are due to damage occurring anywhere between the cortex and L1 in the spinal cord. Since the spinal cord ends at level L1, lesions below this level will not produce UMN signs. Conditions which can lead to UMN signs are listed in Table 7.14.

Although a specific area of the frontal lobes (precentral gyrus) is designated the primary motor cortex (see Fig. 7.12), many neurones from other areas of the cortex are also involved in planning and initiating conscious movement and so can also be called upper motor neurones. This includes neurones of both descending tracts. Damage to the descending tracts will produce the same effects as damage to the neurones themselves.

## Observation

Damage to the corticospinal neurones and tracts will result in contralateral loss of skilled movements. Lack of movement will in turn eventually lead to a form of muscle atrophy known as disuse atrophy. Damage to the multineuronal pathway causes release of inhibition on the LMNs in the spinal cord, especially those which innervate the antigravity muscles, producing the effect most commonly associated with UMN lesions, that of spasticity or stiffness in the limbs.

**Gait.** Observation of the patient's gait is an important part of the assessment for UMN lesions. In the lower limb the effect is extension at

**Table 7.14**  Conditions associated with UMN signs

- Cerebral palsy due to anoxia at birth
- Cerebral vascular accidents
- Brain injury
- Friedreich's ataxia
- Spinal injury
- Brain or spinal tumours
- Amyotrophic lateral sclerosis (motor neurone disease)
- Vitamin $B_{12}$ deficiency
- Multiple (disseminated) sclerosis
- Later stages of syringomyelia

the hip and knee, with plantarflexion and inversion of the foot. If the effect is unilateral, the person is described as hemiplegic. The inability to flex the knee and hip leads to a circumductory gait, with the lateral border of the forefoot and toes often scraping the ground. If both sides are affected the person is paraplegic and the gait is described as a scissor gait, with the knees adducted and feet abducted. Walking aids such as Zimmer frames are essential.

## Clinical tests

**Clasp-knife spasticity.** The affected limb will be initially stiff to passive stretch, but if gentle stretch is continued, the limb may suddenly relax, rather like the opening of a clasp-knife. This is due to a length-dependent inhibition of the stretch reflex (see Fig. 7.16).

**Tendon reflexes.** Due to the reduced inhibition by the multineuronal tracts, the alpha LMNs responsible for the contraction of extrafusal fibres are hyperexcited. This results in exaggerated patella and ankle tendon reflexes and clonus – increased rhythmic contractions elicited at the ankle or patella by causing brisk stretch of the muscles. More than three contractions as a result of testing the patella or Achilles reflex is indicative of UMN damage (Fuller 1993b).

**Plantar reflex.** Damage to the corticospinal neurones or their axons has another effect that is clinically detectable, the so-called plantar reflex or Babinski sign. It has been suggested that the abnormal reflex, a dorsiflexing big toe, is due to release of a spinal inhibitory reflex (Van Gijn 1975). The plantar surface of the foot is stroked firmly and briskly from the posterolateral border of the heel to the hallux as shown in Figure 7.17. The normal response is a slight plantarflexion of the hallux and lesser toes, although no response is also often seen, especially in the elderly where the sensory pathway may be affected. In patients with corticospinal tract dysfunction, the hallux will extend (dorsiflexion of the hallux) and the lesser toes may fan out. This is the extensor response, sometimes referred to as a positive Babinski response. However, the normal response does not become established until the

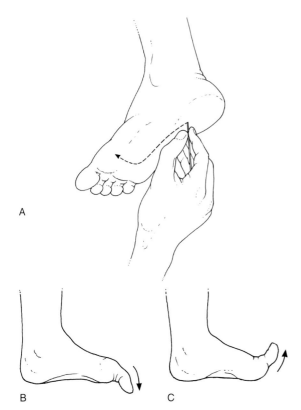

**Figure 7.17** The Babinski response **A.** Eliciting the response **B.** Flexor response (normal response) – toes plantarflex **C.** Extensor response (positive Babinski sign) – toes dorsiflex.

person has learnt to walk and so an extensor response is quite normal in babies. It is important not to rely only on this test for diagnosis of UMN lesions as it is easy to elicit a pain withdrawal response which may appear similar to an extensor response. The rest of the clinical picture should also suggest UMN lesions.

**Muscle tone.** Due to the release of spinal inhibition in UMN conditions, the LMNs will be in a hyperexcited state and so will be firing more frequently. This will result in greater muscle 'tone' and the affected muscle will feel very firm or tense.

Any condition which causes damage to the UMNs or their descending tracts can produce UMN signs. If the cortex is affected, the effects will occur on the contralateral side of the body, and if the lesion is in the spinal cord, the effects will be on the same side, below the level of the lesion (Case history 7.1).

*Hospital tests*

The use of tests to diagnose UMN lesions will vary according to the suspected cause. For example, brain scans are indicated if a CVA is suspected, whereas a spinal radiograph would be used if a tumour of the spine was suspected.

## Lower motor neurone lesions

As the lower motor neurone cell body, its efferent fibres, the neuromuscular junction and the 10–600 skeletal muscle fibres it innervates all act as a coordinated whole, damage to any part of this motor unit will produce similar effects of weakness (paresis) or complete loss of function (paralysis) and reduced or absent reflexes. Diseases principally affecting the muscles are called myopathies, but this can be confusing as often the cause is lesions in the LMN which have given rise to atrophy of the muscle. Therefore, assessment of all parts of the motor unit will be considered in this section. For classification of myopathies, see Table 7.15.

Since LMNs or their spinal nerves exit at all segments of the spinal cord, LMN symptoms can be seen as a result of damage to any segment from

---

**Case history 7.1**

A 70-year-old female Caucasian presented to the clinic complaining of excessive wear on the lateral border of the left shoe and a corn on the dorsum of the fifth toe. The patient walked with a stick and had a slow, circumducted gait; the left arm was held in a flexed position.

Neurological assessment revealed normal tendon reflexes and muscle power in the right leg but exaggerated tendon reflexes and an extensor plantar response (positive Babinski sign), clonic spasm of the muscles and signs of muscle atrophy in the left leg.

**Diagnosis:** History taking revealed the patient had suffered a major CVA, which had affected the right cortex. The clinical features were consistent with the history. Fortunately for the patient she was right-handed so her speech was not affected and she was still able to feed herself and write.

**Table 7.15** Classification of myopathies

| Classification | Descriptor |
| --- | --- |
| Inherited | Muscular dystrophies (at present untreatable) <br> Duchenne's – X-linked recessive condition. Commonest and most serious of the inherited dystrophies. Affects males, females are carriers. Onset before age 10 years. Weakness in proximal and girdle muscles of lower limb first, later upper limbs also. Hypertrophy and later fatty infiltration (pseudohypertrophy) of calf muscles. Cardiac muscle also affected. See ele vated levels of serum phosphokinase. Death from respiratory failure usual between 20 and 30 years <br> Becker's – X-linked recessive condition. A more benign variety of the above <br> Dystrophia myotonica – autosomal dominant condition. Gene located on chromosome 19. Insidious onset, usually between 20 and 50 years, but can be present earlier. Progressive weakness and wasting of distal as well as proximal limb muscles, facial and sternomastoids. Cardiomyopathy, cataracts and frontal baldness also common. Myotonia is failure of muscle to relax immediately after contraction. Patient cannot open hand quickly after making a fist. Faulty gene leads to defective chloride ion transport, resulting in membrane hyperexcitability <br> Facio-scapulo-humeral-autosomal dominant condition – benign, often asymptomatic. Wasting and weakness of facial, scapular and humeral muscles mean patient has difficulty in whistling, heavy lifting, etc., as well as scapula in abnormal position <br> Limb girdle – variable inheritance (may be treatable, depending on cause). Several causes: specific biochemical defect, benign form of motor neurone disease, polymyositis, hormonal and metabolic disease |
| Biochemical defect | McArdle's syndrome. Abnormality of glycogen metabolism due to deficiency of muscle phosphorylase. Patient suffers from fatigue, cramps and muscle spasm. <br> Malignant hyperpyrexia. No muscle wastage or weakness. Symptoms occur during or immediately after administration of a general anaesthetic, especially if halothane or the muscle relaxant suxamethonium chloride is given. Defect in calcium metabolism gives rise to prolonged muscle contraction, in turn raising body temperature. Fatal in 50% of cases |
| Acquired inflammatory | Polymyositis-autoimmune disease. Infiltration of monocytes and muscle necrosis. Weakness of proximal limb, trunk and neck muscles. Patient has difficulty raising hands above head, getting up out of low chairs and bath. May be associated pain on muscular exertion <br> Dermatomyositis. As above, with additional involvement of skin of face and hands, with erythematous rash |
| Non-inflammatory | Secondary to high-dose steroids and thyrotoxicosis. These are the most usual causes, but can also be associated with alcoholism, Cushing's disease, Addison's disease, acromegaly, osteomalacia and malignancy. See weakness of proximal limb muscles and shoulder girdle. Trunk may also be involved |

C1 to S5. However, due to the anatomy of the spinal cord any damage to the cord from L2 will only result in an LMN lesion. It is possible to see a combination of UMN and LMN symptoms if the lesion is between C1 and L1, e.g. syringomyelia. The conditions that can lead to lower motor neurone lesions are listed in Table 7.16.

## Observation

If the pathway is interrupted or damaged in any way, either at the level of the cell body or along

**Table 7.16** Conditions associated with lower motor neurone lesions

- Poliomyelitis
- Injury to lower motor neurone and/or peripheral nerve
- Motor neurone disease
- Syringomyelia
- Vitamin $B_{12}$ deficiency
- Cord compression/lesion (Brown–Séquard syndrome)
- Spina bifida
- Charcot–Marie–Tooth disease

---

**Case history 7.2**

A 54-year-old male Caucasian first presented to the clinic complaining of corns and callus under the metatarsal heads of both feet. He was unable to bend down to cut his toe nails.

A vascular assessment revealed weak pulses in both feet, with the right foot being cold. A neurological assessment revealed dimished reflexes in the right leg and absence of vibration sense in the right foot. Two-point discrimination was 2 cm in the left foot and 10 cm in the right foot. Orthopaedic examination showed a leg length discrepancy of 2.5 cm, the right leg being the shorter and having developed a functional equinus at the ankle. Muscle wastage was apparent in the lower limb of the right side. The patient walked with a limp.

**Diagnosis:** The signs and symptoms are all consistent with poliomyelitis. The patient had contracted the virus when a child. The lower motor neurones of the right side of the spinal cord at the level of the lumbar plexi had been affected.

---

**Case history 7.3**

A 52-year-old Caucasian female presented to the clinic with plantar callus and fissuring, which had arisen following plantar fasciotomy to correct 'clubbed feet'. The patient stated that she had been born with normal feet, but by the time she was 6 years old she could not run or jump properly and by the time she was an adolescent her feet had become high-arched and inverted.

She had noticed a gradual weakness in her arms and legs and on one accasion, when 41 years old, she had almost dropped a baby while working as a nursing auxiliary. This incident had caused her to be sent for a neurological examination which revealed slowed motor nerve conduction velocities. She had a recent history of several falls, with her ankle 'going over'. She also complained of aching joints in the feet, knees and hips. Her 27-year-old son was similarly affected.

Neurological examination showed all sensory perception except vibration to be normal, but reflexes were absent. Muscle power was reduced in all limbs and muscle wasting of hands, feet and calf muscles was noted. Orthopaedic examination showed reduced dorsiflexion and eversion, with a pes-cavus-type foot and high-stepping gait.

**Diagnosis:** The patient suffered from Charcot–Marie–Tooth disease, also known as peroneal muscle atrophy. It is an inherited peripheral neuropathy and exists in more than one form, the two most common forms being autosomal dominant.

---

its axon, then the impulse cannot reach the muscle. The result will be weakness (paresis) or flaccid paralysis, depending on the site and extent of the damage. The sites of damage may involve:

- lower motor neurone, e.g. poliomyelitis virus (Case history 7.2)
- peripheral axon, e.g. diabetes mellitus
- neuromuscular junction, e.g. destruction of cholinergic receptors of the skeletal muscle as in myasthenia gravis.

Myopathies will also produce weakness or paralysis, even if the lower motor neurone is intact.

In contrast to UMN lesions, which affect particular movements, LMN lesions and myopathies affect particular muscles (Case history 7.3). For example, if the tibialis anterior nerve is affected the anterior tibial muscle is unable to control deceleration of dorsiflexion at the ankle in gait, producing a characteristic slapping gait (Root et al 1977).

Nerve impulses are essential to the health of the muscle, so that lack of impulses leads to much more rapid atrophy of muscle, skin and other soft tissue than seen in UMN lesions. This is known as denervation atrophy. In addition, the denervated muscle becomes highly sensitive to very small amounts of neurotransmitter (acetylcholine), possibly due to upregulation of receptors. This results in a quivering of the muscle (fasciculation), seen on an electromyogram as fibrillation. This effect will not be seen if the lesion is in the muscle itself.

*Clinical tests*

**Muscle power:** Muscle power can be graded according to the Medical Research Council scale (Fuller 1993c) as follows:

5  = normal power
4+ = submaximal movement against resistance
4  = moderate movement against resistance
4– = slight movement against resistance
3  = moves against gravity but not resistance
2  = moves with gravity eliminated
1  = flicker
0  = no movement.

A reduced strength of contraction suggests paresis or paralysis.

**Fatiguability.** If the site of the lesion is the neuromuscular junction, the muscle will show a sliding decrease in response or fatiguability as seen in myasthenia gravis. The acetylcholine receptors are destroyed in an autoimmune attack and although the first quanta of neurotransmitter can diffuse to remaining receptors, subsequent release of neurotransmitter is less and less likely to make contact and so the response fades. The muscle cells are able to replace the receptors but the autoimmune attack will strike again, in the same or different muscles.

**Muscle tone.** In the skeletal muscles of a healthy person there will always be some motor units firing, which means that the muscle will feel firm. This is referred to as the 'tone' of the muscle. In LMN or muscle damage, the muscle will feel flabby, because of loss of this tone.

**Tendon reflexes.** Reflexes will be weak or absent, because of interruption of the final common pathway. A single reduced or absent reflex suggests mononeuropathy or radiculopathy. A reduction or absence of all lower limb reflexes suggests polyradiculopathy, cauda equina lesions, peripheral polyneuropathy or a myopathy. In the latter there will be no sensory deficit.

### Hospital tests

Again, the tests selected vary according to the suspected cause. For example, if diabetic polyneuropathy is suspected, the diagnosis could be confirmed by a combination of sensory testing, nerve conduction tests and blood glucose measurements.

**Nerve conduction.** To measure motor conduction velocities the stimulating electrode is placed along the path of the nerve and the recording electrode is placed over the belly of the muscle. Amplitude and duration of the action potential are also recorded. The lower limit of normal conduction velocities in the lower limb is 40 m/s.

Nerve conduction tests, whether sensory, motor or mixed nerve, do not give definitive diagnoses but help to confirm diagnosis: e.g. by comparing the affected side with the healthy side as in diagnosing tarsal tunnel syndrome (Galardi et al 1994) or by distinguishing between axonal degeneration and segmental demyelination, the two chief pathological processes occurring in peripheral nerve diseases. The distinguishing characteristics are shown below.

Axonal degeneration, e.g. the polyneuropathies of diabetes mellitus, alcoholism, toxicity due to heavy metals, nerve entrapment and Friedreich's ataxia (Zouri et al 1998):

* see clinical changes first (weakness, numbness, atrophy)
* slowing of nerve conduction velocities and loss of large fibres
* reduction in action potential amplitude
* more prominent distally than proximally (longest fibres affected first)
* fibrillation seen on electromyograph.

Segmental demyelination, e.g. vasculitis of rheumatoid arthritis (acquired, chronic), Guillain–Barré syndrome (acquired, acute/chronic), Charcot–Marie–Tooth disease/peroneal muscular atrophy/hereditary motor and sensory neuropathy (inherited, chronic):

* electrophysiological changes seen first
* dramatic fall in nerve conduction velocities, maybe even total conduction block
* worsens proximally.

Charcot–Marie–Tooth disease is interesting because two subtypes have been identified: HMSN type I, which shows primarily segmental demyelination, and HMSN type II, which shows mainly axonal degeneration (McLeod & Lance 1989b).

**Electromyography.** This uses a needle electrode inserted into the muscle to show the electrical activity of the muscle in response to an electrical stimulus. Abnormal results are detected in dysfunction of motor nerves, neuromuscular junction lesions and in myopathies (Matthews & Arnold 1991). Electromyography is the only means of electrophysiological testing for myopathies:

* if due to motor nerve denervation (e.g. poliomyelitis), will see reduced recruitment,

**Table 7.17** Differences between upper motor neurone and lower motor neurone lesions

| Upper motor neurone | Lower motor neurone |
| --- | --- |
| Exaggerated tendon reflexes | Loss of tendon reflexes |
| Extensor plantar response (positive Babinski sign) | Flexor plantar response (negative Babinski sign) |
| Loss of abdominal reflex | Normal abdominal reflex |
| Normal electrical excitability of muscle | Fasciculation (fibrillation seen on EMG) |
| Some muscle wasting over a period of time due to lack of use | Marked muscle wasting occurs relatively quickly |
| Increase in muscle tone (clonus) | Flaccid muscles (lack of tone) |
| Whole limb affected | Certain muscle groups affected depending on site of damage; deformity due to contracture of antagonists |

fibrillation, then a reduction in nerve action potential amplitude
- if due to changes at the neuromuscular junction (e.g. myasthenia gravis), will see a reduction in recruitment
- if due to muscle disease (e.g. Duchenne's muscular dystrophy), will see spike potentials on the electromyograph.

Tests may be performed that are specific to particular conditions, such as detection of the presence of antibodies to cholinergic receptors in myasthenia gravis.

**Nerve and muscle biopsies.** These are obtained in an identical manner to those described for sensory nerve biopsies. Histological examination of nerve and muscle tissue will show structural abnormalities, and biochemical tests will detect enzyme dysfunction: e.g. in distinguishing Duchenne's muscular dystrophy from the treatable connective tissue disease of polymyositis, which also shows muscle weakness and atrophy of limb girdles.

The differences between UMN and LMN lesions are summarised in Table 7.17.

## ASSESSMENT OF COORDINATION/PROPRIOCEPTION FUNCTION

The receptors in the muscles, joints and tendons all feed position sense information to the cerebellum and cortex. In turn, the cerebellum and the cortex bring about vital postural reflexes and reflexes necessary for accurate movement. The basal ganglia also play an important part in the coordination of movement. Damage to these parts of the nervous system may have an effect on gait and coordination. Conditions that may affect coordination and proprioception function are listed in Table 7.18.

## Observation

Careful observation of motor activity can give an indication of a deficit in posture, balance or coordination; for example, a stamping gait may be due to loss of proprioception as occurs in

**Table 7.18** Conditions that may result in poor coordination

| Part | Conditions |
| --- | --- |
| Cerebellum | Tumour<br>Multiple sclerosis<br>Arnold–Chiari malformation<br>Friedreich's ataxia<br>Other hereditary spinocerebellar ataxias<br>Hypothyroidism<br>Repeated head trauma as in boxing |
| Basal ganglia | Parkinsonism<br>Huntington's chorea<br>Wilson's disease<br>Sydenham's chorea |
| Ascending pathways | Subacute combined degeneration of the spinal cord<br>Guillain–Barré syndrome<br>Tabes dorsalis<br>Alcoholism |

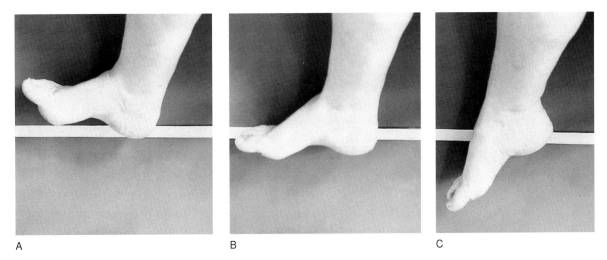

A B C

**Figure 8.2**   Sagittal plane motion at the ankle   **A.** Dorsiflexion: movement of the foot toward the anterior aspect of the tibia   **B.** Neutral position   **C.** Plantarflexion: movement of the foot away from the tibia.

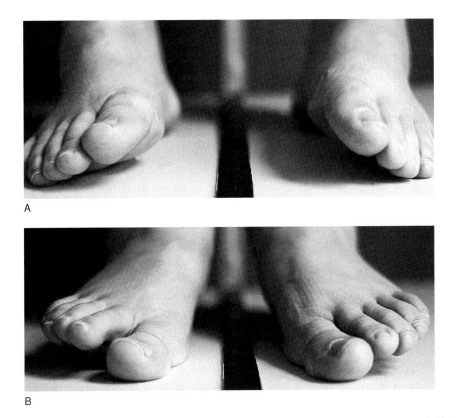

A

B

**Figure 8.3**   Frontal plane motion in relation to the midline of the body (black line)   **A.** Inversion: the foot is lifted up and away from the line   **B.** Eversion: the foot is moved down and towards the line.

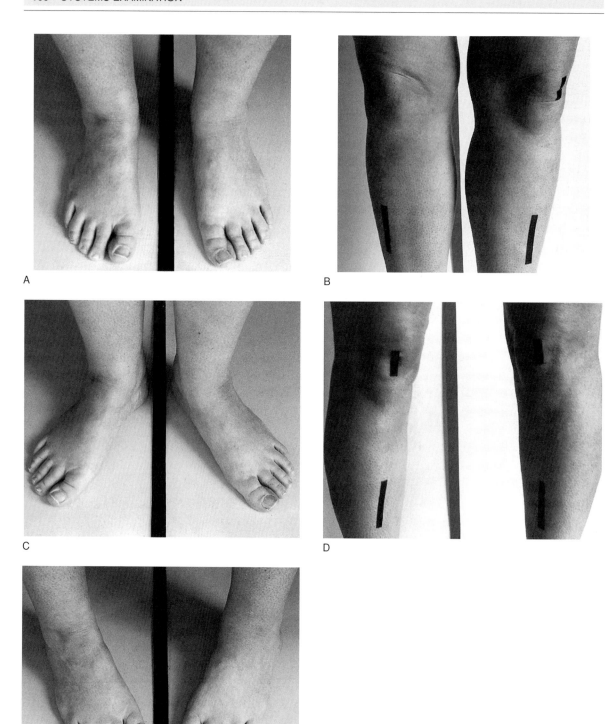

**Figure 8.4** Relationship between transverse plane motion in the leg and transverse plane motion in the foot **A.** The feet are mildly abducted; this is the normal standing position **B.** The legs are externally (laterally) rotated, which results in abduction of the feet (**C**) **D.** The legs are internally rotated (medially), which results in the adduction of the feet (**E**).

foot the use of the terms *adduction* and *abduction* is dependent upon the site of the reference point: the midline of the body or the midline of the foot. Functionally, the midline of the body is usually used as the reference point: *abduction* of the foot is where the distal part of the foot moves away from the midline of the body and *adduction* when the distal part of the foot moves towards the midline of the body (Fig. 8.4). Anatomically the midline of the foot is commonly used as the reference point: e.g. adductor hallucis is inserted into the lateral side of the proximal phalanx of the hallux and is so termed because it brings about adduction of the hallux – movement of the hallux towards the midline of the foot.

**Triplanar motion.** The position of the joint axis together with the shape of the articulating surfaces can result in joint motion in more than one plane. If a joint axis is positioned at an angle of less than 90° to all the cardinal body planes triplanar motion occurs – *pronation* and *supination*. *Pronation* is the collective term for dorsiflexion, eversion and abduction and *supination* for plantarflexion, inversion and adduction. In the foot the subtalar and midtarsal joints produce triplanar motion.

## Position of a joint

To describe the position of a joint the suffix -ed is used:

* *sagittal plane* – extended and flexed (thigh and leg); dorsiflexed and plantarflexed (foot)
* *transverse plane* – internally and externally rotated (thigh and leg); adducted and abducted (foot)
* *frontal plane* – abducted and adducted (thigh and leg); inverted and everted (foot)
* *triplanar* – pronated and supinated (foot).

It is important that a distinction is made between joint motion and position; a joint moves in the opposite direction to the position it is in. For example, at heel-strike the foot is slightly supinated (position) but as soon as the heel contacts the ground pronation (motion) occurs at the subtalar joint in order to absorb shock from ground contact.

## Deformity of a part of the body

The term 'deformity' is used to describe a fixed position adopted by a part of the body. Terms used to denote deformity usually have the suffix -us:

* *Sagittal plane* – equinus when the foot or part of the foot is plantarflexed, e.g. ankle equinus, and extensus when the foot or part of the foot is dorsiflexed, e.g. hallux extensus. Calcaneus, although rarely seen, is used to describe the calcaneus when it is in fixed dorsiflexion, e.g. talipes calcaneovalgus.
* *Frontal plane* – varus and valgus (Fig. 8.5).
* *Transverse plane* – adductus or abductus.

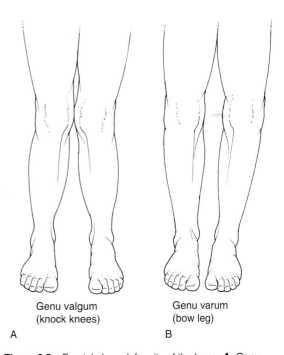

Genu valgum
(knock knees)

A

Genu varum
(bow leg)

B

**Figure 8.5**    Frontal plane deformity of the legs    **A.** Genu valgum (knock knees): the knees are close together and the medial malleoli are far apart    **B.** Genu varum (bow legs): the knees are far apart and the medial malleoli are close together.

**Table 8.1**   Factors that can affect normal function

- Hereditary/congenital problems, e.g. Charcot–Marie–Tooth disease, talipes equinovarus, CDH
- Acute/chronic injury causing pain, e.g. slipped femoral epiphysis, ankle sprain
- Abnormal alignment secondary to trauma, e.g. femoral/ tibial/ epiphyseal fracture
- Abnormal alignment (developmental), e.g. internal femoral torsion, genu valgum
- Infections, e.g. tuberculosis
- Neurological disorders, e.g. CVA
- Muscle disorders, e.g. Duchenne's muscular dystrophy
- Neoplasia, e.g. osteosarcoma
- Systemic disease, e.g. autoimmune (rheumatoid arthritis), bone disease (Paget's disease)
- Degenerative processes, e.g. osteoarthritis
- Joint hypermobility, e.g. Marfan's syndrome
- Osteochondroses, e.g. Perthes' disease
- Psychological factors, e.g. attention seeking
- Footwear, e.g. high-heeled shoes

## WHY IS AN ORTHOPAEDIC ASSESSMENT INDICATED ?

Normal lower limb function should be pain-free and energy-efficient. The main purpose of the assessment is to identify whether the system is functioning within the boundaries of 'normality'. Normal function can be affected by many factors (Table 8.1). It should be remembered that orthopaedic lower limb problems are not always isolated in origin. They may result from referred pain from a proximal source or can be part of a systemic disorder. It is therefore important that the lower limbs are not examined in isolation and that observation and examination of other parts of the body are undertaken where indicated.

In summary the purpose of an orthopaedic lower limb assessment is to:

- establish the main complaint(s), e.g. pain, stiffness, tenderness, numbness, weakness or crepitus
- identify the site of the primary problem – e.g. foot, leg, knee, hip – and try to relate to underlying structures
- identify any secondary problems and relate them to the primary problem, e.g. lesion patterns, pronation due to leg-length discrepancy
- identify the cause of the problem, e.g. abnormal alignment

- establish how the problem evolved
- identify any movement/activity that produces/exacerbates symptoms
- identify movement/activity that relieves symptoms
- establish any differential diagnoses
- utilise the data from the assessment to produce an effective management plan
- utilise the data from the assessment to monitor the progress of the condition.

## The assessment process

When undertaking an assessment of the lower limb it is essential that the system is observed weightbearing (dynamic and static) and non-weightbearing. Differences between the two can help to determine whether compensation has occurred. For example, non-weightbearing assessment may identify the presence of a forefoot varus; observation of the patient's gait may show this problem has been fully compensated through abnormal pronation at the subtalar joint. Conversely, information from the non-weightbearing assessment may explain the cause of a gait abnormality, e.g. a patient may have a bouncy gait due to an early heel lift; non-weightbearing assessment of the ankle joint may reveal that the cause is an ankle equinus due to a short gastrocnemius muscle.

**Foot position/shape.** When all the foot is in contact with the ground the position of the foot in relation to the midline of the body should be observed. Normally the foot should be slightly abducted (approximately 13°). If the foot is adducted (in-toeing) or excessively abducted (out-toeing) this should be noted together with whether the problem is bi- or unilateral. Foot shape can help inform us about function. High-arched cavoid feet (high STJ axis) produce a greater percentage of internal/external leg rotation, which can result in proximal symptoms in the lower limb. In contrast, low-arched flat feet (low STJ axis) produce increased frontal plane motion, which can result in symptoms in the foot (Green & Carol 1984).

**Muscle activity.** The anterior view allows muscle activity to be observed (Fig. 8.10). Normal 'decelerator' muscle activity can be observed. Deceleration implies that the muscle resists joint movement by eccentric contraction; extensor tendons on the dorsum of the foot are active at contact because they decelerate the foot, prevent foot slap and allow the sole to contact the ground smoothly (Fig. 8.8A,B). Paralysis of the anterior muscle group will lead to a rapid collapse of the foot on to the ground and an audible slap. An example of a severe form of muscle group weakness is shown in Figure 8.11. The peronei, longus and brevis are difficult to identify during gait unless they show spasm. When this happens, and it is not common, the tendons stand out around the lateral malleolus (peroneus longus) and lateral foot (peroneus brevis).

**Propulsion.** A lateral view of the first MTPJ at propulsion is useful to check whether the normal range of dorsiflexion (approximately 70°) is achieved. An alteration in gait at propulsion is often seen in hallux limitus/rigidus to avoid painful dorsiflexion. Furthermore, observation of the whole foot is necessary to assess whether a rigid lever is formed at propulsion and that the foot is not propulsing off an unstable hypermobile forefoot (a cause of first ray pathology).

**Swing phase.** The foot pronates during early swing because the STJ provides additional dorsiflexion with pronation to aid ground clearance. Some neuromuscular conditions may

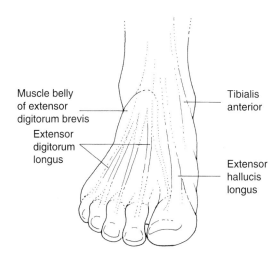

**Figure 8.10** Muscles on the dorsal aspect of the foot. It is important to observe muscle activity during gait. The contraction of the extensor and tibialis anterior muscles should be clearly seen (Fig. 8.8A,B).

prevent this from occurring and lead to the toes dragging across the ground, e.g. poliomyelitis. Signs of skin lesions over the digits may provide a clue that this is happening. Hip flexors and internal rotators contract to bring the leg forward. If the hamstrings are injured, the time spent in the swing phase will be reduced.

## Abnormal gait patterns

Gait can be affected in a variety of ways, leading to abnormal gait patterns. Some of the commonly encountered gait patterns are described below.

**Antalgic gait.** This is usually due to a painful muscle, ligament or joint in the lower limb. Furthermore, a painful superficial skin lesion, e.g. verruca, can cause the patient to alter his gait so as to avoid weightbearing on the painful area of the foot. An antalgic gait may commonly be seen following an ankle sprain (lateral ligaments).

**Apropulsive gait.** During the propulsive stage of gait the MTPJs should dorsiflex to approximately 70° and the hallux should be the last digit to leave the ground; if this does not occur, the gait is said to be apropulsive. An apropulsive gait may occur due to a variety of factors, e.g. hallux limitus/rigidus, abnormal pronation, unusual

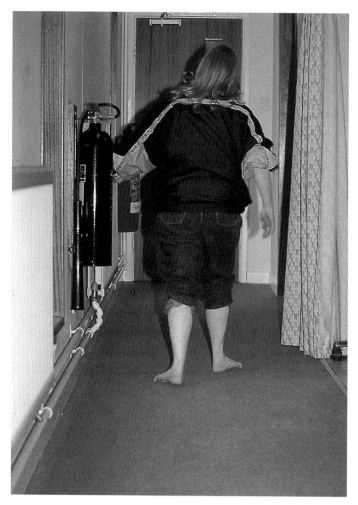

**Figure 8.11** The flat-footed and abducted gait has been brought about by muscle paresis (weakness) in the lower leg. Extensive tests have shown no obvious diagnosis. The gait shows shuffle-waddling. There is marked abduction with bilateral ground contact for most of the stance phase. The left foot shows medial roll off as the leg prepares to move into swing.

metatarsal formula, excessive internal rotation of the leg. The foot may compensate for lack of propulsion by rolling off its medial border (Fig. 8.11), by propelling from a hyperextended (dorsiflexion) first IPJ rather than MTPJ or by an abductory twist. This is when the distal part of the foot twists outwards during propulsion. Whatever the cause, the foot is prevented from re-supinating during the later stages of mid-stance. However, once the heel lifts off the ground the effect of ground reaction, which prevented the re-supination, is reduced and the fore-

foot twists outwards in order to bring the foot into a more medial position for toe-off.

**Abnormal pronation.** Abnormal pronation can be classified as excessive pronation and/or pronation occurring when the foot should be supinating. Signs of abnormal pronation during gait are excessive/prolonged internal rotation of the leg, eversion of the calcaneus, abduction at the midtarsal joint, an apropulsive gait and abnormal phasic activity of the muscles.

**Early heel lift.** This may vary from the heel making no contact with the ground (toe walking) to a relatively normal heel contact but an early heel lift. Heel lift should normally occur at the end of midstance prior to propulsion. An early heel lift can give rise to a bouncy gait. The most common cause is an ankle equinus.

**Limb-length inequality (LLI).** One shoulder is usually lower than the other, and there may be a functional scoliosis. The determinants of gait are affected and the gait appears uneven. The foot of the shorter leg is usually in a supinated position and the foot of the longer leg abnormally pronates. Early heel lift may occur in the shorter leg and prolonged flexion of the knee of the longer leg.

**Trendelenburg gait.** This is characterised by a lurching/waddling gait where the pelvis tilts to the affected side. Associated with congenital dysplasia of the hip and hip osteoarthritis (due to weak gluteus medius), Trendelenburg gait can present following Achilles tendon lengthening procedures and will remain as long as posterior leg muscle weakness persists.

**Painful knee joint.** Avoidance of extension.

**Painful hip joint.** It is commonly held in slight flexion, abduction and external rotation because this puts least stress on the capsule or inflamed synovial membrane. Walking speed and time spent on the involved hip is reduced, e.g. osteoarthritis, Perthes' disease and slipped capital femoral epiphysis.

**Foot drop or steppage gait.** A high knee lift is produced during gait to ensure ground clearance of the affected limb. It is often associated with peroneal damage (Charcot–Marie–Tooth disease), weak tibialis anterior or poliomyelitis.

**Circumducted gait.** A CVA victim has the characteristic features of unilateral limb weakness and will circumduct (rotate the leg in an arc) and flex the elbow and hand towards the body. Movements are made slowly to maintain balance. Jerky movements suggest muscle coordination problems; the nature of upper and lower motor neurone deficits are described in Chapter 7.

**Scissoring gait.** The legs cross the line of progression during gait in cerebral palsy. Circumduction is necessary in order to produce forward motion.

**Dystrophic/atrophic gait.** An exaggerated alternation of lateral trunk movements with an exaggerated elevation of the hip suggestive of the gait of a duck or penguin is seen in Duchenne's muscular dystrophy (Sutherland et al 1981).

**Festinating gait.** Small accelerating shuffling steps are taken often on tip-toe. This gait pattern is typically associated with Parkinson's disease.

**Ataxic gait.** This condition produces an unstable poorly coordinated wide base of gait pattern. It is primarily seen in patients with cerebellar pathology.

**Helicopod gait.** The feet describe half-circles as they shuffle along during contact and early midstance phase. This condition is seen frequently in hysterical disorder.

## NON-WEIGHTBEARING EXAMINATION

The prime purpose of the non-weightbearing examination is to undertake an assessment of the joints and muscles of the lower limb. Information from this part of the examination may explain the cause of a gait abnormality or the patient's presenting problem. For example, a foot may in-toe as a result of an osseous and/or soft tissue problem of the leg; the purpose of the non-weightbearing examination is to establish which is most likely.

A flat couch is required for the patient to lie on. The patient should feel comfortable and relaxed and should not wear restrictive clothing.

Non-weightbearing examination involves an assessment of the following:

- hip
- knee
- ankle
- subtalar
- midtarsal
- metatarsals
- metatarsophalangeal joints (MTPJs)
- digits (proximal and distal interphalangeal joints – IPJs)
- alignment of the lower limb.

### Hip examination

The hip joint is both a mobile and stable joint. Stability is provided by the depth of the acetabulum, strong capsule, capsular ligaments and surrounding muscles. Mobility occurs in all three body planes.

The primary presenting problem is often hip pain (coxodynia). This is felt deep in the groin, whereas pain on the outside of the femur is often referred pain from the spine. A hip problem can occasionally result in pain being referred (via the obturator nerve) to the knee. A patient who cannot accurately localise pain in the knee should be suspected of having a disorder of the hip. The main cause of hip pain is osteoarthritis, a particularly common condition in the elderly. An X-ray of the hip should be considered if confirmation of a disease process is necessary or diagnosis unclear, e.g. osteoarthrosis, Perthes' disease.

It is not usually necessary to examine every patient's hip. The hip should only be examined if the patient complains of discomfort or pain in the area and/or gait analysis reveals an abnormality which affects normal pelvis and thigh/leg motion.

Observation of the hip for gross deformity, muscle wasting, oedema, contusion and scar will provide valuable information about potential or past pathology. In addition, palpation of the hip region for joint, muscle pain/tenderness or bursitis (e.g. greater trochanter bursitis due to overuse, weakness of gluteus medius on the opposite side or LLI) is helpful. Where a hip examination is indicated, a series of tests on the hip joint itself in addition to the muscles acting upon it is undertaken.

### Hip joint tests

Assessment of hip motion should be undertaken in each of the three body planes – sagittal, frontal and transverse.

**Sagittal plane.** To ensure forward progression during gait, sagittal plane motion at the hip is necessary. Ideally, there should be approximately 120–140° of flexion and 5–20° of extension, although not all of this is necessary for gait. To assess hip flexion the patient is placed supine on a firm, flat couch. The practitioner holds the leg firmly and flexes the hip by pushing the leg towards the body until resistance is met (Fig. 8.12). To assess extension the patient is placed in the prone position. The practitioner places one hand on the posterior superior iliac crest to stabilise the

pelvis while the other hand holds the opposite leg just above the anterior knee and moves the leg towards the body to the point of resistance.

Loss of sagittal plane motion may be due to pain, femoral nerve entrapment or effusion in the hip joint as the anterior ligaments (iliofemoral and pubofemoral) will be under greater tension and resistance than usual. Any asymmetry should be noted.

**Frontal plane.** To assess abduction and adduction at the hip the patient lies supine and the practitioner holds the leg just below the anterior knee. The leg with the knee extended is moved across the opposite leg (adduction) and then brought back and abducted. The pelvis should be stabilised during this assessment by placing a hand on the opposite iliac crest. There should be less adduction than abduction at the hip. Tightness of the adductors on abduction can lead to a scissors-type gait: this is when one or both legs have a tendency to cross over during gait and can be seen with cerebral palsy.

**Transverse plane.** Internal and external rotation of the lower limb is essential for normal gait. Ideally, the total range of transverse plane motion in an adult should be 90°, comprising 45° internal and 45° external rotation. Females tend to show more internal rotation than males (Svenningsen et al 1990). The range of transverse plane motion at

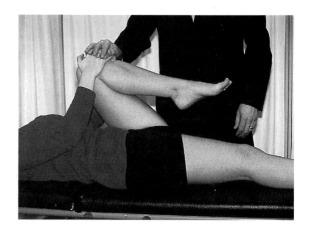

**Figure 8.12** The patient should be asked to draw the leg towards the stomach as depicted in the photograph. The hip is flexed to its limit against the abdomen. Thomas's test should be considered at the same time by looking for contralateral lifting.

the hip decreases with age and the DOM changes from symmetry to more external than internal rotation.

To assess transverse plane rotation the patient lies in a supine position. The hip and knees are flexed and the leg is moved medially and laterally as one would the arms of a clock. A gravity goniometer can be used to assess the range of motion (Fig. 8.13). Asymmetry in the DOM should be noted. For example, a patient who shows 70° internal rotation and only 20° external rotation has an internally rotated femur which will affect normal lower limb function and may result in abnormal pronation at the subtalar joint.

The test can be repeated with the patient in the same position but with the hip and knees

extended. The practitioner may note a difference in the ROM and DOM at the hip when the knees are flexed compared to when they are extended. It was thought that this technique could be used to detect the presence of torsion (bone influence) or version (soft tissue influence). Torsion was said to exist if there was no difference between the ROM and DOM at the hip with the knees flexed and extended and version if there was a greater ROM when the knees were flexed. It was considered important to make a distinction as torsion cannot be treated conservatively while version can. This concept, while plausible, is not consistent with bone torsion measurement and is open to misdiagnosis. However, it is important when

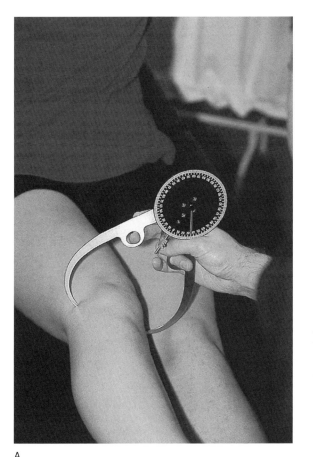

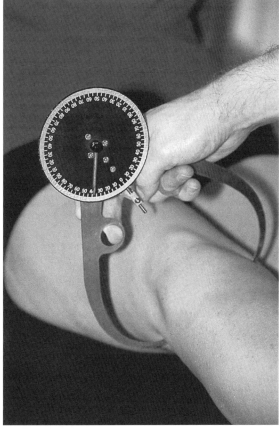

A

B

**Figure 8.13**   The hips are in a flexed position   **A.** A gravity goniometer is used to assess the amount of internal femoral rotation   **B.** A gravity goniometer is used to assess the amount of external femoral rotation.

undertaking an assessment of the muscles around the hip to see if there are any soft tissue contractures, which may be responsible for limiting motion. Contracture of capsular structures of the hip will limit hip movement when these structures are on-stretch (hip extended), whereas contracture of the medial hamstrings will limit external hip rotation with the hip in a flexed position.

**Scouring/circumduction test.** This test is used to assess QOM and joint congruency in patients complaining of groin pain. The hip is flexed and adducted and the practitioner rotates the hip to test for any crepitations. If pain is provoked during this manoeuvre with the hip internally rotated a lesion of the acetabular labrum should be suspected. A posterolateral force applied to the hip will test the integrity of the posterior/lateral hip capsule.

**Patrick's or faber's test (*f*lexion *ab*duction *exter*nal *r*otation).** The patient lays supine with one leg straight. The other knee and hip are flexed so that the heel is placed on the knee of the straight leg. The knee is then slowly lowered into abduction. Gentle pressure is applied to the flexed knee while the opposite hand stabilises the pelvis over the opposite anterior superior iliac spine. This test stresses the medial hip capsule by placing an anteromedial force on the hip, the integrity of the iliofemoral/pubofemoral ligaments and also assesses for sacroiliac discomfort.

**Sacroiliac joint provocation test.** Patients who experience pathology of the sacroiliac joint may complain of pain in the region of the hip. It is therefore important to be able to exclude pathology in the sacroiliac joint. To isolate and test this joint the practitioner places her hands on the anterior superior iliac spines of the pelvis and presses down firmly and evenly to compress the joint and stress the sacroiliac ligaments. The test is positive if the patient experiences unilateral pain in the abdominal-groin, gluteal region or the leg.

### Hip muscle tests

**Young's test.** A taut tensor fasciae latae causes the knee and hip to flex. By abducting the lower limb, tension on the tensor fasciae latae is reduced

and any flexion deformity should disappear. A tight tensor fasciae latae may be the cause of an apparent limb length discrepancy.

**Thomas's test.** Iliopsoas consists of psoas major, psoas minor and iliacus (the prime flexors of the hip). Thomas's test is used to rule out the presence of iliopsoas contracture. If a flexion deformity exists the affected leg will flex at the knee (see Fig. 8.12) (Case comment 8.3). Furthermore, the femoral nerve can be irritated by a taut iliopsoas group. Damage to the nerve will lead to weakness of the quadriceps, as well as loss of sensation on the anterior and medial aspects of the leg (Case comment 8.4).

**Ely's test.** This test is used to assess hip flexor (rectus femoris) tightness or contracture. The patient lies prone and the knee is slowly flexed as far as possible until the heel comes close to the buttocks. Observe the buttock/hip during this manoeuvre. The point at which the buttock rises off the couch on the tested side indicates the degree of hip flexor tightness.

**Ober's test.** This test is designed to assess for iliotibial band contraction or tightness. The patient lies on his side and the outer limb with the knee extended is moved anteriorly and then adducted towards the couch (Fig. 8.14A). This stretches the lateral structures, primarily the

---

**Case comment 8.3**

Thomas's test: while the patient flexes the hip, the practitioner must observe the opposite (contralateral) thigh for any sign of elevation. The lumbar spine must lie flat. If the iliopsoas muscles are tight, the contralateral hip will rise as the ipsilateral hip will force the lumbar spine against the couch. Fixed flexion will cause an apparent LLI.

---

**Case comment 8.4**

The obturator nerve arises in the psoas major and crosses the hip joint, exiting through the obturator foramen. If this nerve is injured in the hip region, e.g. due to a slipped capita femoris epiphysis, knee pain may result. Where knee pain exists, hip pathology must always be ruled out.

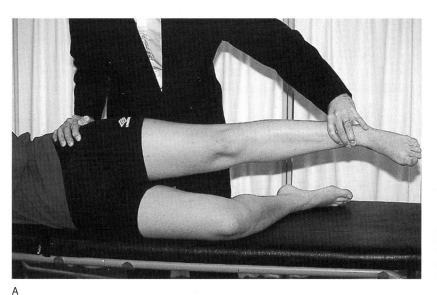

A

**Figure 8.14** **A.** Ober's test identifies resistance in the tensor fascia/iliotibial tract
**B.** Assessment of the external rotators. Muscle strength can be gauged by resisting external rotation **C.** The patient is asked to bring the knees together against resistance. This tests adductor strength.

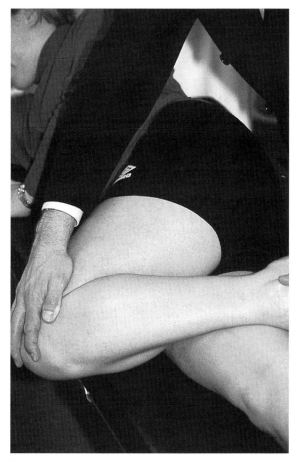

B

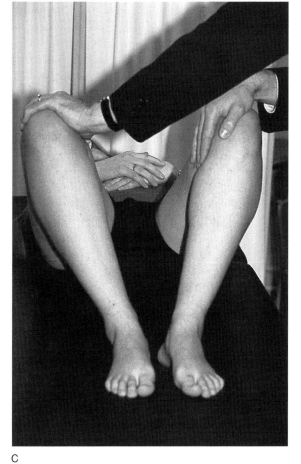

C

iliotibial band. A modified form of the test separately tests the short fibres of the knee; this is achieved by flexing the knee and repeating the manoeuvre.

**Piriformis test.** With the patient lying on his side, the hip and the knee are flexed to 90°. The examiner places one hand on the pelvis for stabilisation and with the other hand applies pressure at the knee, pushing it towards the couch. This puts the piriformis muscle on tension. If tightness of the piriformis muscle is impinging on the sciatic nerve, pain may be produced in the buttock and also down the leg. Also, in this position the strength of the external rotators of the hip can be tested by asking the patient to externally rotate the hip against resistance (Fig. 8.14B).

**Adductor strength test.** The adductors have their insertion on the medial side of the femur along the linea aspera. The adductor muscles are important during the swing phase, stabilising the contralateral side of the hip against the pelvis as the leg swings forward. Adductor strength can be tested as in Figure 8.14C. Gracilis, a partial adductor, rotates the femur on the hip. As it shares some of the function of the adductors, it can be examined with them. However, this muscle crosses the knee and lies between the sartorius and semitendinosus on the medial aspect of the knee. The knee should be extended to include the action of gracilis, but flexed to remove its influence.

**Abductor strength test.** The abductors include the gluteus medius and minimus as well as tensor fasciae latae. Together they act through the iliotibial tract. Abductor strength is best assessed when the subject lies on his side. The patient should raise the upper leg away from the couch against gravity and resistance.

**Trendelenburg's test (Stork test).** This tests the stability of the hip and the ability of the hip abductors to stabilise the pelvis on the femur. The patient stands on one leg with the other knee flexed; the pelvis should tilt upwards or stay level on the side of the lifted leg. A positive Trendelenburg sign occurs when the reverse happens: the pelvis tilts downwards, indicating weak glutei. Osteoarthritis of the hip can produce a positive Trendelenburg sign.

**Lasèque's (straight-leg-raise) test.** This test will provoke pain in patients with hamstring muscle inflexibility, severe hip pathology and also tests mobility of nerve roots L4 to S2. Where no pathology is present the leg should make an angle of 70° to the supporting surface (Gajdosik et al 1993, Kendall et al 1993). There is no significant difference in hamstring flexibility between males and females (Gajdosik et al 1990).

*Functional tests*

If the patient's pain has not been reproduced during formal examination, then functional tests should be performed. A single leg squat can be used to assess pelvic control. Abnormalities of excessive lateral or anterior tilt may be noted. Step-up or step-down tests may also be useful.

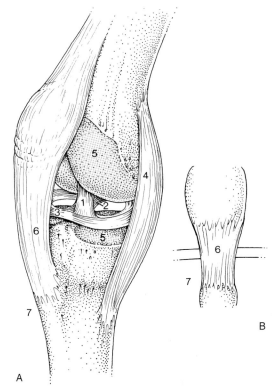

**Figure 8.15A,B    A.** Normal knee anatomy:    **(1)** anterior cruciate    **(2)** posterior cruciate    **(3)** meniscus    **(4)** collateral ligament    **(5)** cartilage    **(6)** ligamentum patellae surrounding patella    **(7)** tibial tubercle    **B.** Diagrammatic representation of the joint margin.

## Knee examination

The knee joint is the largest joint in the body. It is a complex structure which is comprised of the patellofemoral and tibiofemoral joints. The knee should be examined if dysfunction is observed during gait and/or the patient complains of knee discomfort/pain. To make a comprehensive assessment of knee function a detailed history is required. It is important that the practitioner establishes whether knee pain/discomfort is due to a primary problem affecting the knee, e.g. meniscus tear, or to compensation for a problem elsewhere, e.g. abnormal pronation causing instability and damage to the knee.

Figure 8.15 illustrates the anatomy of the knee joint and the knee joint margin. The knee joint can be compared to a boiled egg lying on a plate; the configuration of an oval femoral surface on a flat tibial plateau allows great mobility. During gait it is important that the knee is stable; the cruciate and collateral ligaments, the menisci and the iliotibial band and sartorius muscles provide most of the stability.

The patella forms part of the knee joint; it articulates with the anterior surface of the inferior

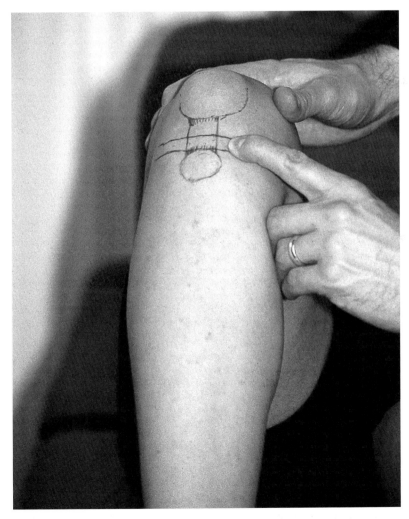

C

**Figure 8.15C**  Photograph of the joint margin corresponding to **B**. (Fig. 8.15A,B on facing page.)

end of the femur. It acts as a sesamoid as described earlier and provides a key mechanical advantage, increasing the moments of force applied through the ligamentum patellae on to the tibial tubercle.

The history should be followed by a comprehensive clinical examination of the knee joint and its associated structures. In view of the number of structures involved, assessment needs to be approached in a systematic manner. The key feature of the knee examination is that each structure that may be injured must be examined. The following scheme of assessment is suggested:

- observation
- palpation
- patellofemoral joint tests
- tibiofemoral joint motion
- tibiofemoral joint stability
- integrity of internal knee structure
- muscle testing
- Q angle
- functional tests
- laboratory tests.

## Observation

Prior to formal examination the knee should be observed for:

- Gross deformity (genu valgum/varum, enlarged or abnormal position of tibial tubercle).
- Patellar position (squinting, fisheye or outward facing, patella alta, patellar tilt or rotation).
- Patellar size (small patella unstable in femoral groove, susceptible to subluxation/ dislocation).
- Oedema – the presence and site of swelling in the knee should be noted (Case comment 8.5). Swelling of an extreme nature can be associated with bursitis, acute synovitis, tearing of the menisci, rheumatoid arthritis (Baker's cyst) or osteoarthritis. Spontaneous swelling is usually caused by cruciate or meniscus injury or haemarthrosis following trauma.
- Tonic muscle spasm (hamstrings) secondary to intra-articular/extra-articular pain.

---

> **Case comment 8.5**
>
> A 10-year-old male developed a tender area on the anterior aspect of his knee during activity. The site of the tibial tubercle was shown to have been damaged by force from the traction of ligamentum patellae, leaving clinically a hot swollen prominence. The condition was Osgood–Schlatter's disease, a common example of a traction apophysitis. Examination may reveal an old unilateral or bilateral condition typified by an enlarged tubercle.

- Muscle wasting (quadriceps femoris, particularly vastus medialis). Often associated with anterior knee pain, osteoarthritis, rheumatoid arthritis and Osgood–Schlatter's disease.
- Bruising (trauma).
- Scars (site and size will provide evidence of type/extent of surgery).

## Palpation

Systematically palpate the knee to localise areas of pain/tenderness and thereby isolate the structures involved:

- Palpate for warmth (inflammatory joint disorder).
- Palpate for oedema (generalised/localised).
- Palpate joint line medially/laterally for joint, meniscal pathology and anteriorly for coronary ligament pathology.
- Tendons crossing the knee joint: medially (semitendinosus/semimembranosus); laterally (biceps femoris, iliotibial band); and anteriorly (patellar tendon).
- Patellar: tenderness superior pole (rectus femoris tear or bipartite patella); pain in body of patellar (fracture following trauma); pain inferior pole of patellar (Sinding–Larsen–Johansson syndrome); infrapatellar fat pad palpated for tenderness – this fat pad can become impinged between the patellar and femoral condyle following forced extension of the knee (Hoffa's syndrome); however, chronic fat pad impingement (aka infrapatella bursitis) occurs more frequently.

the medial border of the tibia can be associated with medial tibial stress syndrome. Tenderness over the inferior tibiofibular joint may be associated with lateral ligament injury and may cause anterior ankle pain. Tenderness in the back of the calf may be associated with a ruptured plantaris tendon syndrome, whereas pain over the tendo calcaneus may be suggestive of a partial or complete rupture. With the patient prone, Thomson's test can be performed. The calf is squeezed. If no ankle plantarflexion occurs, a complete rupture is indicated.

The frontal plane alignment of the tibia should be determined because tibial deformity can influence foot function. This is best performed in the supine position by bringing the legs together and observing the relative distance between the knees and malleoli. A greater distance between the knees is seen in tibial varum. Tibial varum is generally more common than tibial valgum. In the largest normative study, Astrom & Arvidson (1995) reported a mean of 6° of tibial varum; therefore, a slight tibial varum is considered normal. An excessive tibial varum, however, can lead to a range of lower limb conditions with the development of pathology theoretically dependent on the STJ's ability to compensate. Unilateral overuse injuries are more likely to exhibit larger tibial varum on the affected side (Tomaro 1995).

The eight-finger test can also be used to estimate the degree of frontal plane bowing of the tibia. All eight fingers are placed along the anterior border of the tibia and their alignment compared. Sagittal plane bowing (sabre tibia) and general tibial thickening as seen in Paget's disease should not be overlooked (Fig. 8.19). It is also important to assess for any transverse plane deformity of the tibia, as this can influence foot function. Medial tibial torsion is associated with flat feet and intoeing deformities (Thackery & Beeson 1996), whereas a lateral torsional deformity of the tibia is seen in pes cavus. With the patient supine and knees flexed and the soles of the feet on the couch, the relative lengths of the tibiae should be assessed by comparing the heights of the knees (Skyline/Allis test) or tibial tuberosities.

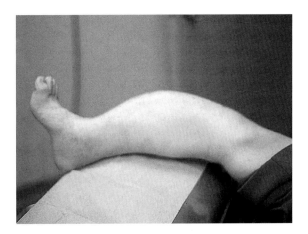

**Figure 8.19**    Patient with severe bowing associated with Paget's disease, 'sabre tibia' affecting patients in the sixth/seventh decade of life. Deformity occurs in the sagittal as well as the frontal plane.

## Ankle examination

Inman (1976) regards the ankle as a two-joint system comprising the talocrural joint (TCJ) and the subtalar joint (STJ). Motion of the foot is primarily controlled through this joint complex, but the whole proximal segment also relies upon the TCJ and STJ working in concert. Elftman (1960) considered the midtarsal joint to be the third member of the ankle complex. In addition, Brukner & Kahn (1993) consider the inferior tibiofibular joint to be part of the ankle joint complex. The inferior tibiofibular joint is a syndesmosis supported by the inferior tibiofibular ligament. A small amount of rotation is present at this joint. Each of these joints will be considered separately for examination purposes but functionally they should be considered together.

Coalitions between the joints making up the ankle complex may be present. The two most common involve the talocalcaneal (medial and posterior facets) and the calcaneonavicular (Kulik & Clanton 1996). Other types may occur but are quite rare. The coalition may be fibrous, cartilaginous or osseous. Fibrous coalitions permit some motion whereas cartilaginous and osseous coalitions produce little motion but more symptoms. Tonic spasm of the peronei is a common finding with tarsal coalitions. X-rays are necessary to diagnose a synostosis (osseous coalition).

*Talocrural joint*

The trochlear surface of the talus articulates with the inferior surface of the tibia to form the talocrural joint. The medial and lateral malleoli provide additional articulations and stability to the ankle joint. The talocrural joint is a triplanar joint but, because of the position of its axis and the shape of the joint surfaces, its main motion is in the sagittal plane. The lateral curvature and radius of the trochlear surface of the talus has been found to be variable – the longer its radius, the less dorsiflexion (Barnett & Napier 1952). During midstance there should be at least 10° of dorsiflexion at the ankle in order to allow the leg to move over the foot.

The body compensates for a lack of ankle dorsiflexion at the knee and/or subtalar and midtarsal joints. The STJ has less available sagittal plane motion than the TCJ, but if necessary the STJ will increase the amount available if there is insufficient motion at the TCJ. In addition, the knee can hyperextend (genu recurvatum) as a way of compensating for an ankle equinus.

Assessment of TCJ range of motion, stability, strength, palpation for tenderness, grading of ligamentous injury and proprioception are important parts of the ankle joint assessment.

**Joint motion.** The passive range of TCJ plantarflexion and dorsiflexion should be assessed and compared for each limb. Ankle equinus is traditionally defined as less than 10° of dorsiflexion at the TCJ, although some practitioners suggest that less than 5° dorsiflexion leads to abnormal compensation. It may arise from soft tissue or bone abnormalities of an acquired or congenital nature.

Assessing sagittal plane motion at the TCJ is difficult. It can be assessed either weightbearing or non-weightbearing. If assessed non-weightbearing the patient should lie in a prone or supine position with the knee extended and the foot and ankle free of the end of the couch. The practitioner holds the foot in a neutral position with one hand, places the other hand on the sole of the foot and dorsiflexes the ankle (Fig. 8.20A). If subtalar joint pronation is allowed to occur during the examination a falsely elevated

dorsiflexion value will result (Rome 1996a, Tiberio et al 1989).

The force applied by the practitioner to produce TCJ dorsiflexion can vary; this will have an effect on the result. A tractograph can be used to assess the range of motion but the practitioner may find it difficult to use, while at the same time keeping the foot in a neutral position (Fig. 8.20B). In addition the intra- and interobserver reliability of non-weightbearing TCJ dorsiflexion measurements using a tractograph is questionable (Rome 1996b).

A tight soleus and/or gastrocnemius may prevent TCJ dorsiflexion. To differentiate between the two the amount of dorsiflexion with the knee extended and flexed should be measured. With the knee flexed the tendons of gastrocnemius which cross the knee are released from tension and as a result a tight gastrocnemius should not affect TCJ dorsiflexion. If the amount of dorsiflexion is still reduced when the knee is flexed the cause is likely to be soleus (Fig. 8.20C). A bony block (osteophytes on distal/anterior tibia) can also limit TCJ dorsiflexion with the knee flexed; however, the tendo Achilles in this case will feel slack.

Assessment of the TCJ end-of-ROM is useful. Soft tissue limitation will result in a springy endfeel, whereas limitation resulting from a bony block will be abrupt.

More consistent results have been achieved when sagittal plane motion is assessed with the patient weightbearing. The patient stands facing a wall with a distance of approximately 0.5 m between the patient and the wall. One leg, with the knee in a flexed position, is placed in front, approximately 30 cm from the wall. The other leg is placed behind the forward foot with the knee extended and the foot held in a neutral position. The patient leans towards and places both hands on the wall and is asked to move his body towards the wall. In order to do this the patient must dorsiflex the ankle of the limb furthest from the wall. The amount of dorsiflexion can be measured with a tractograph (Fig. 8.20D).

**Stability.** By moving the TCJ in all three planes the ligaments can be stressed and any tenderness noted. There should be little or no

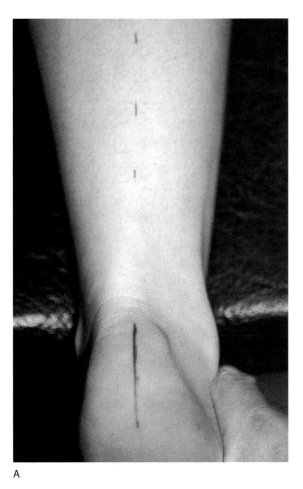
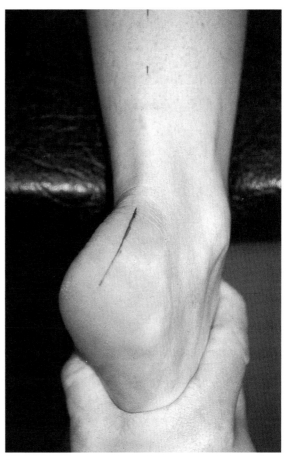

A                                                                          B

**Figure 8.22**    Assessing frontal plane motion at the STJ    **A.** The distal third of the leg is bisected and a line is drawn at the bisection point. The posterior surface of the calcaneus is moved into its maximally everted position and the angle between the bisection of the leg and the bisection of the calcaneus is measured    **B.** The calcaneus is moved into its maximally inverted position and the angle between the bisection of the leg and the bisection of the calcaneus is measured.

- inverted forefoot
- everted forefoot.

For treatment to be effective it is important that the cause and the extent of the abnormal pronation are correctly identified; otherwise, only symptomatic treatment on a trial and error basis can be provided.

### Examination of muscles affecting the ankle complex

**Plantarflexors.** The posterior group of muscles plantarflex the foot at the ankle but may also restrict the amount of dorsiflexion at the ankle.

The patient should be asked to plantarflex the foot with and without resistance in order to test muscle strength. Rupture or partial rupture of the tendo Achilles should be ruled out. If the tendo Achilles is functioning normally the foot should plantarflex when the calf muscle is squeezed. Plantaris is a small muscle that is not present in everyone. Spontaneous rupture of plantaris may occur; it shows as a painful medial swelling over the posterior aspect of the calcaneus at its insertion near the tendo Achilles.

**Invertors.** Tibialis posterior and anterior are the main invertors of the foot. These extrinsic muscles play an important role in re-supinating the foot during midstance and propulsion. To assess the strength of these muscles the patient should be asked to move his foot into supination against resistance.

**Dorsiflexors.** The main dorsiflexors of the foot are the long extensors and tibialis anterior. To assess the strength of the anterior muscles the patient should be asked to dorsiflex the ankle with the foot in inversion against resistance. Weakness of the anterior group is often linked to neurological problems, e.g. poliomyelitis. The plantarflexors have a work capacity 4.5 times that of the dorsiflexors. If the dorsiflexors are weak the foot is held in a plantarflexed position as the plantarflexors have a mechanical advantage.

**Evertors.** The evertors of the foot are the peronei. To assess the strength of the peronei the patient should be asked to evert the foot against resistance. The evertors are not as powerful as the invertors and in the case of neurological problems and/or muscle imbalance the invertors have a mechanical advantage over the evertors and the foot is held in an inverted position (following a CVA). Tonic spasm of the peroneal muscles can occur; this is noted particularly with tarsal coalitions. A local anaesthetic can be administered in order to differentiate between a muscle spasm and a tarsal coalition.

## Midtarsal joint

The MTJ comprises two synovial joint complexes: talonavicular and calcaneocuboid. The MTJ is also known as the transtarsal or Chopart's joint, and is an articulation between the rearfoot and forefoot. The MTJ has two axes: longitudinal and oblique. The longitudinal axis provides frontal plane motion facilitated by the ball and socket joint of the talonavicular articulation. The oblique axis involves both calcaneocuboid and calcaneotalonavicular joints and primarily produces transverse and sagittal plane motion. Limitations of motion at the ankle joint are compensated at the oblique axis of the MTJ.

The MTJ assists in reducing impact forces and helps to prepare the foot for propulsion. It can also accommodate walking on uneven terrain

without affecting the rearfoot. This means that the forefoot might invert while the heel remains vertical; the converse does not occur.

**Joint motion.** To assess the motion at the MTJ the practitioner must stabilise the STJ and prevent any motion occurring at this joint by firmly holding the heel with one hand and holding the foot just distal to the midtarsal joint with the other. The MTJ should then be moved in the sagittal, transverse and frontal planes. There should be most motion in the sagittal and transverse planes and minimal motion in the frontal. The position of the axes will affect the amount of motion at the MTJ: e.g. a high (vertical) oblique axis will result in an increase in transverse plane motion but a reduction in sagittal plane motion.

## Metatarsal examination

The first and fifth metatarsals have independent axes of motion and produce triplanar motion. The second metatarsal is firmly anchored to the intermediate cuneiform and has least motion; the third has less motion than the fourth metatarsal. Whereas the first and fifth metatarsals provide triplanar motion, the central three only move in the sagittal plane. The ability of the first metatarsal to plantarflex is important in order that the medial side of the foot makes ground contact during gait and the first MTPJ can dorsiflex during propulsion. Patients commonly present with cutaneous changes associated with dysfunction of the metatarsals, especially the first and fifth. Sometimes one of the metatarsals may be held in a plantarflexed position. The position of the metatarsals can subsequently affect foot mechanics and gait.

**Joint motion.** Clinical assessment of first and fifth metatarsal motion can only be satisfactorily undertaken in the sagittal plane. Unlike most joints, motion at the first and fifth rays is measured in millimetres, not degrees. To assess sagittal plane motion the patient can be in a supine or prone position. The feet must be allowed to hang free of the couch. The practitioner places one hand, with the thumb to the plantar surface, around the lateral side of the forefoot including the second metatarsal while maintaining the foot

Case comment 8.6

It should be remembered that a patient who has had a discrepancy for years will have compensated by altering his/her body posture. If any raise under the heel is considered, this must only be for a proportion of the difference. Heel raises used alone may cause unwanted plantar flexion, especially when the deformity is greater than 2.5 cm. The adaptation to footwear should affect the whole sole in this case.

- foot supinated on the short side
- foot pronated on the long side
- knee flexed on the long side
- ankle plantarflexed on the short side.

Limb length measurement is only performed if the patient's symptoms or dynamic function suggest that a discrepancy may be present.

To assess for the presence of a real LLI the patient lies supine on a flat couch with the hips and knees extended. The practitioner places her hands around the heels and exerts a slight pull on the legs, at the same time bringing the legs together so that the knees and malleoli are touching. The knees and malleoli should be level. A difference indicates an inequality at the femur or tibia. To identify which bone is affected the knees should be flexed and the heels pushed flush against the buttocks (Skyline/Allis test) (Fig. 8.32). If the tibiae are of unequal length, the knees or tibial tubercles will be at different levels. If one femur is longer than the other, the knee of the longer femur will be positioned further forward than the other knee. This is a relatively crude method of assessment and does not quantify the extent of the difference.

A flexible non-stretch tape measure with a metal end can be used to measure a real leg length ('direct measurement technique'). With the patient supine the distance between the anterior superior iliac spine (ASIS) and the medial malleolus is measured (Crawford Adams & Hamblen 1990). The metal end of the tape fits snugly in front of the ASIS, as shown in Figure 8.33A. The practitioner may use any part of the medial malleolus as a reference point, but it is important that the same point is used for repeat measurements. An error of up to 10%

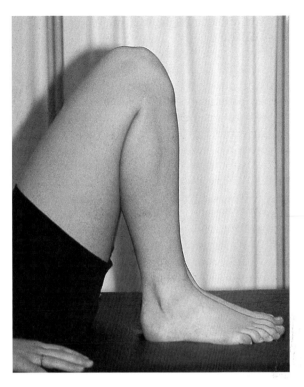

**Figure 8.32** Assessment of leg-length inequality. The knees are flexed so that the position of the knees and ankles can be compared.

should be allowed for because the tape measure may wrap around asymmetrical muscle bulk or, more commonly, the patient's pelvis may not be properly aligned. In cases of asymmetrical muscle bulk, measuring from the ASISs to the lateral malleoli is advocated. A tape measure can be used to compare the individual lengths of the femurs by measuring from the greater trochanter to the lateral knee joint line. The lengths of the tibiae can be compared by measuring from the medial knee joint line to the medial malleolus or the tibial tubercle to the middle of the anterior ankle. The 'indirect measurement technique' can also be used to assess a real leg length. The patient stands while blocks of wood of varying thicknesses are placed under the suspected shorter limb until the iliac crests are palpated to be level.

Radiological measurement (Scannergram) is only used when surgical correction is planned, as it is expensive and, unless the results are going to be used for surgery, exposes the patient to needless radiation.

Distinction between a real or apparent difference can be achieved by measuring each limb from a common reference point above the pelvis; the xiphisternum is usually used. The metal end of the tape is placed on the xiphisternum and the distance from the xiphisternum to each malleolus is measured with the patient (Fig. 8.33B). If values are the same, then the LLI is likely to be apparent. The cause usually lies at the hip or pelvis, where a fixed deformity makes the limbs appear unequal so that the body compensates by tilting laterally. An alternative method can be used with the patient weightbearing:

- The patient stands in the RCSP position (Fig. 8.29A).
- The position of the ASISs is assessed to see if they are level.
- The feet are then placed in the NCSP (Fig. 8.29C).
- The position of the ASISs is assessed to see if they are level.
- If the ASISs are not level in either the RCSP and NCSP, and the extent of the discrepancy remains the same in RCSP and NCSP, a true LLI should be suspected. If the ASISs are on the same level in the NCSP but differ for the RCSP, an apparent LLI should be suspected.

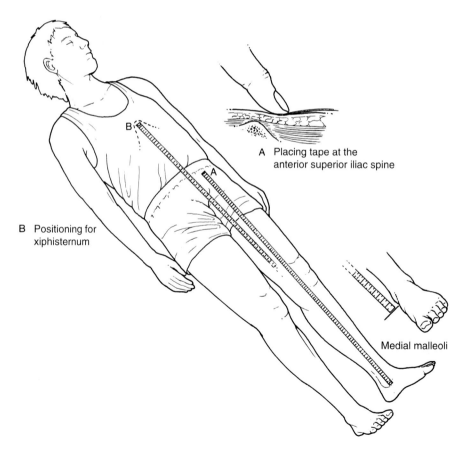

A  Placing tape at the anterior superior iliac spine

B  Positioning for xiphisternum

Medial malleoli

**Figure 8.33**  Assessment of a true and apparent leg-length inequality  **A.** Measurement from the anterior superior iliac spine (ASIS) to the medial malleolus  **B.** Measurement from the xiphisternum to the medial malleolus.

disease is very much dependent on the type of infection and so will be considered accordingly.

## Viral

**Verrucae.** Verrucae (Plate 20) are the predominant viral infection on the foot caused by infection of the skin with human papilloma virus (HPV). Around 5% of 16 year olds will have warts at any one time (Williams et al 1991). The virus affects the stratum spinosum and causes hyperplasia and formation of a benign tumour. Typically, the plantar wart is found under a point of high pressure, e.g. the metatarsal heads or a bony prominence (Glover 1990). In its early stages it appears as a small, dark, translucent puncture mark in the skin. More mature lesions show thrombosed capillaries, a 'cauliflower-rough' surface and are painful when pinched. The patient may complain of increased discomfort on starting to walk after a period of rest, e.g. first thing in the morning. Different types of HPV cause different wart lesions, e.g. flat, genital or plantar.

Verrucae protrude above the level of the skin unless they occur on weightbearing surfaces. When they are found on weightbearing surfaces they protrude into the skin and, as a result, are more painful. Mosaic warts are made up of multiple, small, tightly packed individual warts and may not be painful, whereas plantar warts may be single or multiple and are usually painful. Occasionally, periungual warts may develop around the nail edge and lead to distortion of the nail plate.

Verrucae can usually be diagnosed from their clinical appearance; however, they can be confused with corns (particularly neurovascular or fibrous) and foreign bodies. Verrucae can occur on non-weightbearing and/or weightbearing areas of the foot, unlike corns and most foreign body injuries, which tend to occur solely on weightbearing areas. There may be multiple verrucae present, not only on the feet but also on the hands, the pinching of which tends to cause a sharp pain, whereas corns and foreign bodies give rise to pain on direct pressure. Verrucae appear encapsulated and the skin striae are

broken; corns do not appear encapsulated and the skin striae are not broken but pushed to one side. Any wart with an atypical appearance, particularly in the elderly or immunosuppressed, should be biopsied as, rarely, the lesion may undergo malignant change.

**Molluscum contagiosum.** This is a contagious infection (usually of children) which usually involves the trunk but can affect the leg and foot. Infection with the causative poxvirus, usually by close contact, leads to a papular lesion, which may range in size from a pinhead to a pea. The hard, shiny pedunculated lesion has a central crater from which cheesy material may be expressed by pinching it. The uniqueness of this lesion makes the diagnosis straightforward.

**Herpes zoster (shingles).** Shingles is a recrudescence of previous chicken pox, usually along a single dermatome. It can occur at any age, but most frequently in the elderly or immunosuppressed. It presents as a 1–3-day history of pain or burning in one limb followed by haemorrhagic blisters and later superficial ulcers. Pain may persist for many weeks and months.

**Herpes simplex.** Herpes simplex (cold sores) rarely affect the lower leg, although they may involve the thigh in rugby players (scrum pox) following infected oral exposure to an eroded area of skin on the sports field.

## Bacterial

Bacterial superinfection, which is very common particularly in the various forms of eczema, was discussed earlier. Primary bacterial infections are less common (Plate 21). In all these conditions, full assessment by bacterial swabs is essential.

**Ecthyma.** This infection affects the full thickness of the epidermis. The main pathogens are *Staphylococcus aureus* and *Streptococcus pyogenes*. The patient may have recently been to a humid climate or had an insect bite. It presents as a shallow ulcer with a thick, crusted top.

**Cellulitis.** Cellulitis or erysipelas is a serious infection usually of the lower leg caused most commonly by *Streptococcus pyogenes*. It presents as a flu-like illness that is rapidly followed by a painful red advancing area, usually on the lower leg. The affected area becomes swollen and the skin discoloured. The skin may even blister, necrose and ulcerate. Commonly, a 'portal of entry' is found such as tinea pedis (see below) or a fissured patch of eczema.

**Pitted keratolysis** (Plate 22). Bacterial overgrowths on the sole of the foot secrete proteolytic enzymes that produce multiple pits within the epidermis. The pathogens are microaerophilic diphtheroids. This is particularly common in patients with sweaty feet or who wear trainers. Usually it is asymptomatic, but sometimes the skin thins sufficiently to be tender. Odour is commonly offensive in such patients.

**Erythrasma.** This bacterial infection of creases and flexures occurs between the toes of the foot. It is commonly mistaken for tinea pedis. The pathogen is *Propionobacterium minutissimum*. The skin is usually macerated and red/brown in colour. Again, it has a strong odour and fluoresces coral pink in Wood's light.

## Fungal

There are four patterns of fungal infection of the foot (tinea pedis). Asymmetry is a feature common to all subtypes. In all situations, scrapings are essential to fully assess for fungal disease. Interdigital scaling is the commonest form, usually presenting as itching and fissuring. This usually occurs between the third to the fifth toes where the skin is most macerated. The rash initially begins on one foot, only later extending to the other toes, nails and other foot. A variety of fungi and yeasts are implicated.

**Extension onto the dorsa of the foot** (Plate 23). In chronic disease, the fungus can spread onto the dorsa of the foot, producing itchy scaly rings with an active edge. Fungal culture will help differentiate this from discoid eczema. Typical fungal causes include *Trichophyton rubrum* and less commonly *Epidermophyton floccosum*.

**Blistering in the instep.** The inflammatory reaction on the sole to fungus tends to produce blistering (*Trichophyton mentagrophytes*). It is usually unilateral. Removal of the blister roof will allow closer inspection and it may be sent for culture.

**Moccasin foot.** The soles of the foot can be generally involved with fungus (*Trichophyton rubrum*), producing thickened scaly feet. Often the disease affects both feet. The nails may also be involved. Most patients are unaware of the problem but will have a previous history of infection.

**Onychomycosis.** Tinea pedis may progress to the toe nails (onychomycosis), typically as a result of repeated trauma (e.g. from footwear). Infection may occur superficially on the nail plate or subungually invading under the hyponychium. Proximal subungual involvement occurs rarely in immunocompromised patients or following chronic paronychia. Total nail involvement and dystrophy may result.

**Tinea incognito.** Misdiagnosis of fungal infection is a problem as often the incorrect diagnosis made is eczema. The use of topical steroids to reduce inflammation consequently allows the unsuspected fungus to grow unchecked by the immune system. Patients present with a history of a persistent rash, usually on the foot, which fails to respond to steroid creams. The potency of the steroid used is often very high. The rash is red, ill-defined with nodules within, that when squeezed express pus. Scrapings confirm the presence of fungus (Case history 9.3).

## INFESTATIONS AND INSECT BITES

**Scabies.** The mite *Sarcoptes scabiei* causes scabies. Itching is often severe despite sometimes having minimal evidence of infestation. Patients may describe itchy nodules or blisters. They will usually have family members presenting at the same time with itch. The signs are generally that of eczema but blisters and excoriations are more pronounced. The primary lesion is the burrow of the mite. It appears as a linear or serpiginous white line with scaly opening at one end and a minute grey or red dot at the other end (the mite). The mite may be extracted with a needle and examined using a microscope. Scabies should be suspected in any patient with a pronounced itch, and other sites of involvement (hands and trunk) should be sought.

Case history 9.3

Philip was a 25-year-old footballer who presented with a 4-year history of a troublesome right great toe nail. He was concerned, as the nail was discoloured and growing abnormally. A brief examination of the toe nail suggested fungal disease. Philip explained that since playing professionally he commonly developed a blackened nail on his right foot but recently the colour of the nail had changed and become crumbly. He also mentioned that from time to time he had athlete's foot but had never sought treatment for this. Initially, when asked what medication he was on, he said none; then he remembered that he had been using some steroid cream. A friend had given him some that he used rather unsuccessfully, to treat a patch of eczema on the same foot. On closer questioning, it seemed that the cream had initially helped the eczema but each time he stopped the treatment the eczema just came back again.

On examination, the nail was grossly thickened with creamy linear discoloration at the medial margin extending to the proximal nail fold. The ridged nail was detaching itself from the nail bed. The fourth and fifth interdigital spaces on both feet showed scaling and blistering. Examining the right ankle revealed a thickened erythematous scaly plaque within which were inflamed nodules. The area was markedly excoriated. Microscopy of scrapings from the web space and eczematous plaque revealed the presence of fungus. Culture of the toe nail clippings grew the same fungus, *Trichophyton rubrum* (a common fungus affecting the foot).

**Diagnosis**: Fungal nail and web space disease with tinea incognito of the ankle. The whole problem cleared after discontinuing the topical steroid and a 3-month course of antifungal tablets (terbinafine). He was also advised to check the fitting of his soccer boot.

**Insect bites.** A variety of insects will bite the skin, producing itch or painful nodules or blisters on the skin. The lower leg is commonly involved as it is often exposed (biting insects and fleas). Clues to suggest insect bite are grouped lesions, often along a sock or shoe line, and a history of presence of domestic animals or proximity to farms.

**Larvae migrans.** A variety of hookworms that are gut parasites in animals may find themselves in humans. Cats and dogs are the main carriers. The immature form of the parasite penetrates the skin and the larvae migrate under the skin to produce loops and tortuous tracks.

Patients usually complain of itch and blistering, usually contracting the disease on beaches abroad but occasionally in the UK. The pattern of migration makes diagnosis easy. Fortunately, the disease is self-limiting.

## DISORDERS OF THE SUBCUTANEOUS TISSUE

The subcutaneous layer is a layer of primarily adipose (fat) tissue and covers most of the lower limb, particularly the thighs, anterior shins and plantar surface.

**Atrophy.** Atrophy is the most common disorder affecting the subcutaneous layer. It occurs most frequently as a result of ageing and trauma (e.g. heel pad atrophy in long-distance runners and the elderly) or as a result of granulomatous change (panniculitis) around injection sites (typically, diabetic patients using insulin injections). Affected skin becomes depressed and scarring may occur.

**Painful piezogenic papules.** On the plantar surface, around the heels, herniations of fat from the heel pad into the dermis may be evident on standing. As solitary or multiple nodules they may occasionally give rise to heel pain (Shelley & Rawnsley 1968), usually in middle-aged females. Diagnosis is established, as pain will result from direct pressure while standing, but when non-bearing the lesion completely disappears.

**Erythema nodosum.** This is an uncommon eruption affecting the shins presenting as painful nodules on the shins and less commonly the thighs and forearms. The rash starts as painful areas that enlarge into hot, red nodules, which are acutely tender. These then resolve over a matter of weeks. The redness fades and takes on a bruised appearance. The condition is important, as it is often associated with other diseases such as sarcoidosis and a variety of infections.

## SYSTEMIC DISORDERS AND THE SKIN

The skin is an easily accessible structure and may often give clues regarding internal disease.

Typical disorders which may affect the skin include connective tissue and endocrine diseases. Common systemic disorders and their effects on skin are summarised in Table 9.13.

# PIGMENTED LESIONS

Pigmented lesions represent a large part of general dermatological practice; this is also the case on the lower legs. Pigmented lesions arise as a result of a variety of processes, both neoplastic and inflammatory. Close attention to the clinical history and signs will allow distinction between most lesions.

**Freckles or ephelis.** These are probably the most common pigmented lesions seen on the skin. They are most common in those with fair skin who have been exposed to sunshine. Lesions are usually innumerable; they are visible but not palpable and the pigmentation within is usually evenly distributed and is generally slight. Darker freckles can also occur, particularly after prolonged or excessive sun exposure.

**Lentigo.** A lentigo is a lesion where there is an increase in the number of melanocytes within the skin, resulting in a pigmented patch. Lesions usually occur in older patients and usually arise on sun-exposed sites. Again, the lesion is visible and not palpable; it tends to be solitary and the pigmentation within it is usually light and always even.

**Seborrhoeic warts.** These are particularly common, developing with advancing age. They appear as well-defined, rough, warty, slightly raised lesions that have a stuck-on appearance. They usually occur on the trunk and proximal limbs but can arise on the lower leg. They do not develop on the sole. They are always benign but can become inflamed after minor trauma and may be mistaken for malignancy.

**Pigmented naevi.** Moles are collections of pigmented naevus cells (melanocytes) in the skin

**Table 9.13**  Systemic conditions and their associated skin changes

| Condition | Associated skin changes in the lower limb and foot |
| --- | --- |
| Diabetes mellitus | Increased incidence of skin infections (fungal and bacterial), skin stiffening, ulceration (neurovascular), diabetic bullae, necrobiosis lipoidica, granuloma annulare |
| Lupus erythematosus | Erythematous scaly plaques with follicular plugging |
| Systemic lupus erythematosus | Periungual erythema, splinter haemorrhages, onycholysis and leuconychia. On the legs, erythromelalgia and erythema nodosum |
| Dermatomyositis | Periungual erythema with characteristic 'ragged cuticles'. Occasional calcification within the skin |
| Systemic sclerosis/scleroderma | Tight waxy skin with later distal digital atrophy with calcinosis, ulceration and occasionally gangrene |
| Ehlers–Danlos syndrome | Fragile skin with frequent bruising, hypermobility, poor wound healing, typically showing large scars upon the knees |
| Rheumatoid arthritis | Skin atrophy, nodules, vasculitis with periungual infarcts, splinter haemorrhages and onycholysis with longitudinal ridging of the nails |
| Hyperthyroidism | Hyperhidrosis, clubbing, onycholysis, hyperpigmentation, pretibial myxoedema |
| Hypothyroidism | Anhidrosis, leuconychia, pruritus, palmar and plantar hyperkeratosis |
| Acromegaly | Hyperhidrosis, skin thickening, coarse hair |
| Hepatic disease | Clubbing, spider naevi and pruritus |
| Renal disease | Hyperpigmentation or skin yellowing, nail changes – half-and-half nails, onycholysis |
| Reiter's syndrome | Keratoderma blennorrhagica |
| Internal malignancy | Hyperpigmentation, palmoplantar keratoderma, secondary skin tumours, pruritus, nail clubbing, bullous eruptions |

that contain the pigment melanin. The nature of moles will vary enormously depending on how many naevus cells are present, where in the skin they occupy and how pigmented they are: obviously, the greater number of naevus cells there are, the larger and more protuberant the lesion. Lesions that are close to the epidermal surface tend to be red/brown in colour; however, the further down the pigment is in the skin the bluer the colour becomes. In addition, the intensity of the colour will depend upon how much pigment is being produced. Moles are sometimes present at birth; their number increases during life, most commonly in the first two decades but can develop at any age. Moles may become larger and more pigmented with age and occasionally may regress. The clinical appearances of moles are infinitely variable, therefore making classification on macroscopic grounds alone almost impossible; however, they can be defined according to their microscopic appearances and knowledge of these patterns may be useful in the clinical setting.

**Junctional naevi.** Collections of melanocytes along the dermal–epidermal junction, junctional naevi are the usual type of mole for the sole of the foot. In this site the pigmentation usually follows the ridges and troughs on the epidermal markings. They are usually impalpable, the colour is red brown, and is symmetrical. They commonly occur in children and generally 'mature' by melanocytes falling away into the dermis, forming intradermal naevi. Here, the melanocytes have all fallen into the superficial dermis. Often, the naevus cells stop producing pigment and plump up. Clinically, the lesions are therefore protuberant and pale or skin-coloured. They may continue growing in adulthood. Compound naevi have both junctional and intradermal components and therefore share clinical features of both types of lesions.

**Blue naevi.** Melanocytes that have never reached the epidermis and instead have proliferated in the deeper dermis have a blue appearance. These often develop in later life, especially on sun-exposed sites, especially the dorsa of hands and feet and on the scalp. Blue naevi are small (less than 5 mm) and may be slightly raised. They can be differentiated from vascular malformations in that they do not blanch. They are almost always benign.

**Malignant melanoma** (Plate 24). In the assessment of pigmented lesions the potential diagnosis of melanoma should always be considered. There are a number of clinical symptoms and signs that should alert you to the diagnosis (Table 9.14).

Itching is an early and significant symptom that should be sought. Often, it may be the only presenting symptom, particularly where the melanoma is not in general view. There may be a change in the surface of the mole, skin creases may be lost, and hair follicles and pores may disappear. Almost always there will be an increase in the size, shape or thickness of the mole. This occurs over weeks and months and usually is asymmetrical. Colour will change within a mole; pigment can both increase and decrease within the same lesion. Also, as the melanocytes invade deeper into the skin, they may appear blue or even black. Rarely, melanoma may lose all pigmentation, making diagnosis very difficult clinically (although the patient may recall a pre-existing pigmented lesion). Bleeding, the surface of a melanoma may ulcerate, particularly in advanced disease. The tumour may have spread by the time it is picked up; this may be clinically evident with tumours developing along the lines of lymphatic drainage (in transit metastasis), in the draining lymph nodes or at distant sites (for instance presenting as fits, weight loss or shortness of breath).

Melanoma is very rare before puberty and usually occurs in large congenital moles. The

**Table 9.14**  Suspicious signs and symptoms in a pigmented lesion

| Symptoms | Signs |
|---|---|
| Change in sensation | Loss of skin markings |
| Change in size | Irregular margins |
| Change in colour | Irregular pigmentation |
| Change in shape | Bleeding |
| Change in outline | Ulceration |
| New lesion | |

majority of melanomas develop in later life, occurring in fair individuals on sun-exposed sites and most commonly in women on the lower legs. Melanoma may arise on the sun-protected sole of the foot and, as it is hidden from view, it usually presents late. Any unusual lesion on the foot should be suspected, particularly if there is pigmentation (Case history 9.4).

## SKIN TUMOURS

Tumours of the skin need careful assessment, as there will be clues in both history and examination that will lead to accurate diagnosis. Most lesions will be benign, but a small proportion will be malignant (Table 9.15) and therefore life threatening. Early referral of such lesions to a dermatologist can improve prognosis enormously. Points that should be sought in the history are, obviously, site of the lesion, how quickly it is growing, whether there are associated symptoms such as irritation or pain, or whether there are similar lesions elsewhere. Clinical signs that should be recorded are size, shape, surface, colour, outline, temperature and consistency. Dimensions should be recorded in the notes, and where possible the lesion should be photographed.

---

**Case history 9.4**

A middle-aged female patient presented for assessment of her soft corns, which had been troublesome for many years. After taking a history, the feet were examined, revealing trivial disease; however, on her posterior left calf there was a suspicious pigmented lesion. On questioning the patient, she remembered having a mole on her leg for a number of years but apart from occasional minor irritation it caused her no concern. She tended to burn when she was in the sun and had spent the first 20 years of her life living in Florida. She did not have any family history of melanoma. She was otherwise well. On examination the lesion was 1.5 cm in diameter, the pigmentation was varied and the outline irregular. Within the lesion there was a nodule which had become ulcerated. She was referred to a dermatologist, who confirmed the suspected diagnosis of melanoma by an excision biopsy. She remains free from recurrence.

---

**Table 9.15** Principal tumours affecting the lower limb

| Benign | Malignant |
|---|---|
| Dermatofibroma | Bowen's disease |
| Seborrhoeic wart | Basal cell carcinoma |
| Haemangioma | Squamous cell carcinoma |
| Lipoma | Melanoma |
| Clear cell acanthoma | Kaposi's sarcoma |
| Pyogenic granuloma | Porocarcinoma |
| Eccrine poroma | Metastasis |
| Glomus tumour | |

## Benign tumours

**Dermatofibroma.** The lesions are very common, particularly on the lower leg. They are usually symptomless; often the patient is unaware that the lesion is even there. Sometimes they catch when the leg is scratched or shaved. They are felt as firm tethered nodules within the skin, sometimes with a slightly elevated surface. They often have a pigmented halo and for this reason may be mistaken for more sinister lesions. They are always benign.

**Pyogenic granulomas** (Plate 25). These are common vascular proliferations that grow rapidly over a few days or weeks. They usually follow a minor injury. The surface is very easily broken and bleeding may be prolonged and frequent. In time, the lesion develops a surface epithelium that is more resilient, ultimately resembling a haemangioma.

**Eccrine poroma.** These are benign tumours of the sweat duct that arise on the palms and soles, typically in the over-40 age group. They are pink or red, painless and usually 1–2 cm in diameter with a moist surface, surrounded by a moat-like depression. Occasionally, they can undergo malignant change.

## Malignant lesions

**Bowen's disease.** Bowen's disease is squamous cell carcinoma confined to the epidermis only. It is a condition of the elderly, usually pre-

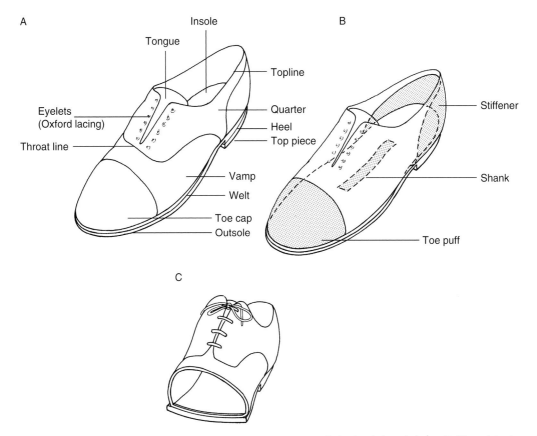

**Figure 10.1** **A.** The 'anatomy' of a lace-up shoe, showing the parts of an Oxford-style laced shoe **B.** The reinforcing within a shoe **C.** Alternative (Gibson) style of lacing.

**Quarter.** The sides and back of the shoe upper are termed the quarters and their top edge forms the topline of the shoe. The medial and lateral sections often join in a seam at the centre of the heel. In lace-up shoes the eyelets for the laces form the anterior part of this section, whereas the tongue is attached to the vamp (Oxford style) or forms part of the vamp (Gibson style, Fig. 10.1C). The inside of the quarter is usually reinforced around the heel by the stiffener. This helps to stabilise the hindfoot in the shoe. In some children's shoes and some athletic footwear the stiffener is extended on the medial side to help resist pronation.

**Toecap.** The upper may have a toecap stitched over or replacing the front of the vamp. It is made into a decorative feature in some men's shoes, for example brogues.

**Linings.** Linings (not illustrated) are included in the quarters and vamps of some shoes to increase the comfort and durability. The lining for the bottom of the shoe is called the insock. It may cover the entire length of the shoe, three-quarters or just the heel section.

**Throat.** The throat is formed by the seam joining the vamp to the quarter. Its position depends on the style of the shoe. A lower throat line, i.e. a shorter vamp and longer quarters, will give a wider/lower opening. This seam will not stretch and therefore dictates the maximum width of foot for which the shoe can be used.

**Insole.** The insole is the flat inside of the shoe which covers the join between the upper and the sole in most methods of construction.

**Outsole.** The outsole or sole is the undersurface of the shoe.

**Shank.** The shank reinforces the waist of the shoe to prevent it from collapsing or distorting in wear. Shanks may not be needed in shoes with very low heels or in shoes where the sole forms a continuous wedge.

**Heel.** The part of the shoe under the heel of the foot, also called the heel, raises the rear of the shoe above ground level. A shoe without a heel or a midsole wedge may be completely flat or have the heel section lower than the forefoot, in which case it is called a negative heel. The outer covering on the surface of the heel, which can be replaced when worn, is called the top piece.

**Welt.** The welt is a strip of material, usually leather, used to join the upper to the sole in Goodyear-welted construction.

## The 'anatomy' of sports shoes

Since trainers replaced plimsolls sports footwear design has developed considerably, bringing new construction methods and terminology to the footwear industry. The functions of sports shoes are different to those of ordinary shoes as, for example, they may be required to absorb shock or provide some medial to lateral stability. The parts of a sports shoe are shown in Figure 10.2 and the terms illustrated are described below.

**Mudguard.** Reinforcing round the outside of the rim of the toe is called the mudguard.

**Saddle.** The saddle is reinforcing stitched to the outside of the shoe in the area of the arch.

**Collar and heel tab.** The topline of a sports shoe is often padded to form the collar. This may be shaped up around the back of the tendo Achilles to form a heel tab. Heel tabs were designed to protect the tendo Achilles but sometimes rub sensitive feet and may therefore need to be removed.

**Hindfoot stabiliser.** One of the elements that may be incorporated into a sports shoe to attempt to counter pronation is the hindfoot stabiliser, which consists of a plastic meniscus between the midsole and the stiffener.

## SHOE CONSTRUCTION
### Lasts

The last is the mould on which most shoes are made and its shape and dimensions will dictate the fit and to some extent the durability of the shoe made on it. It is usually hinged around the instep to allow it to be removed from the shoe when construction is completed. Last design and manufacture are skilled occupations involving the use of many measurements, some of which are shown in Figure 10.3. Most of these are volume measurements rather than the traditional length and width measurements associated with shoe fit. The measurements of the last need to be different from the measurements of the foot to allow for movement in walking and the tightness of fit required by the wearer. It is these factors

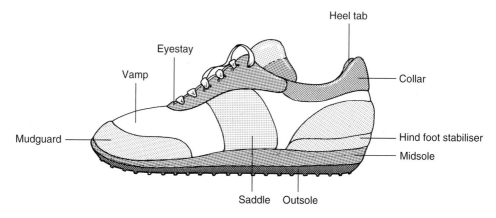

**Figure 10.2**  The parts of a sports shoe.

**Table 10.1**  Points to look for in an ideal shoe

- Laces with at least three eyelets
- Low, wide heel for good stability
- Good width at the front of the shoe to prevent cramping the toes
- Deep, reinforced toe box
- Firm stiffening round the heel
- Curved back for close fit around the heel
- Shaped topline, high enough up the instep for adequate fixation
- Strong leather upper
- Hard-wearing synthetic sole
- Good fit
- Good condition

explanation of why they are important. To assist this task a list of points to look for in a suitable shoe is included in Table 10.1.

## Unsuitable styles of footwear

Mules, clogs and court shoes, the styles on the right of Figure 10.7, are unsuitable for regular wear as they have no means of securing the foot. The only way that mules stay on is by being 'gripped' by the toes. This can lead to toe deformity. Slip-on shoes, especially court shoes, are bought too short and inevitably cramp the toes as the only way that they can stay on the foot is by wedging the foot between the curved back of the heel and the toe puff. When tried on in the correct size the foot slips forward into the toe space and the heel lifts out of the shoe on walking, giving the impression that it is too big. Clogs or slip-on shoes that extend right up the instep will limit forward movement to some extent. A properly fitting lace-up is always preferable (Fig. 10.8).

In most shoes, even 'flat' ones, the heel is raised slightly above the level of the ground, so that the foot is in slight equinus. Even a modest height of heel will tend to throw the weight of the foot forward into the toe section unless it is restricted by an adequate fastening. It is therefore even more important for a high-heeled shoe to have a secure fastening. Raised heels are said to have developed as a protection from dirty streets

but high heels became associated with fashion and style as early as the 16th century. High heels, defined as those that place the foot in more than slight equinus, are not suitable for everyday wear. In addition to the fact that they are nearly always slip-ons, they alter the normal biomechanics of the lower limb in walking. Habitual wear leads to permanent shortening of the calf muscles, barefoot walking is made uncomfortable and in severe cases the heels may not be able to touch the ground.

## ASSESSMENT OF FOOTWEAR

The assessment of footwear should not be seen as a separate entity to be completed after other aspects of the examination but should be integrated into the global assessment. For example, observation of patients walking in their shoes can often be achieved as they enter the clinic and there are some checks of fit which should be done before the shoes are removed. This will ensure that the number of times the shoes need to be removed and replaced is kept to a minimum. Table 10.2 lists the tests that should be included in a simple footwear assessment and

**Table 10.2**  The parts of a simple footwear assessment and the stages at which they can be completed within the global assessment

| Stage of assessment | Test | Brief description |
| --- | --- | --- |
| *In shoes* | | |
| Walking | Observe gait | |
| Standing | Observe stance | |
| | Check length | Palpate end of longest toe |
| | Check heel to ball length | Locate MTPJs in shoe |
| | Check width | Pinch upper over metatarsal heads |
| | Check depth | Palpate toes during flexion |
| *Barefoot* | | |
| Walking | Observe gait | |
| Sitting | History | |
| | Assess suitability of shoes | |
| | Check wear marks | |
| | Examine inside of shoe | |
| Standing | Observe stance | |
| | Note longest toe | |

the stage at which each should be completed. They are described in full below. Performing these checks routinely, as part of a set sequence, will help to ensure that assessment of footwear is completed without undue effort. It should be remembered that hands should be washed between examination of the footwear and the foot. Patients attending for their first appointment should have been warned to bring a selection of their shoes, as new or 'best' shoes may not demonstrate the habitual wear pattern found in the shoes worn every day. There may therefore be several pairs of shoes to examine.

## History taking

Background information about the patient's general footwear and purchasing habits is an essential part of the assessment of footwear.

### Financial circumstances

Before suggesting appropriate footwear, it is important to ascertain the financial circumstances of the patient, as this will influence her ability to follow the advice given. Women tend to spend less per item of footwear than men but they change their footwear more frequently; hence, in total, they spend more on footwear than men (British Footwear Association 1998).

### Wardrobe

Questions regarding the number of shoes owned and the number regularly worn may seem irrelevant but can add helpful information. This line of questioning may uncover that special shoes are worn at work and, therefore, need examination in preference to shoes worn only occasionally. There are specialist reinforced shoes for work in dangerous environments, smart shoes may be needed for office work or special shoes may be required for a specific sporting activity. Advertising and the media influence women's attitudes towards purchasing shoes (Reardon 1999). It is, therefore, important that the practitioner is familiar with current styles within 'the high street' as these could

have a major influence on the style of shoes women are willing to purchase.

### Habits

Details of how often shoes are changed and whether long periods are spent wearing slippers or sports shoes can also be important. For example, a lady is unlikely to benefit from having a pair of suitable shoes to go out in once a week when she spends the rest of the week at home in slippers.

### Acquisition of footwear

Information about when, where and how often patients buy their shoes can be useful: e.g. do they have their feet measured or visit a self-service shop? Whereas 40% of parents start off having their children's feet measured, by the age of 11 years only 15% of children have their feet measured (Stevens 1995).

### Independence

No assessment of footwear would be complete without noting the patient's ability to put on and take off her shoes or to do up and undo the fixation. Many adaptations to footwear and aids to assist independence are available and may form a valuable part of treatment. Sources of information are included in Further Reading.

## Assessment of shoe fit

Shoe fit is always a compromise as the shape of the foot is changing continually due to many different factors, some of which affect length and some girth. The biggest factor affecting length is weightbearing and measurements of length should, therefore, never be made when the patient is sitting. Girth is affected by body weight but is also highly sensitive to both temperature and swelling. There is thus a tendency for feet to be smaller in the morning than the evening. Measurements taken during the middle of the day will give the most representative results.

Assessment of shoe fit is not an exact science: often observation and common sense are all that is required to decide whether shoes fit correctly. Sometimes a method of measuring fit is useful to demonstrate to patients that their shoes are inadequate. A well-fitting shoe should fit snugly around the heel and the arch and allow free movement of the toes.

This section includes a comprehensive list of tests for different aspects of fit. It is not intended that all the tests described should be included in each assessment. They are listed partly to demonstrate the range of potential tests, but also to allow selection of an appropriate test to suit the problems experienced by the patient. In most cases the simplest test described will be adequate but, occasionally, when more accuracy is required, the more complicated measurements can be useful.

The style of the shoe will to some extent dictate fit: e.g. a court or slip-on shoe is likely to be too small in length, width and depth. Additionally, the style of the front of the shoe can have a direct bearing on the fit in this region. Demonstration of poor fit by some of the tests described may help to convert the patient to sensible shoes.

If shoes are really comfortable they are probably a good fit. Strangely, comfort is not as important a factor as might be expected when shoes are being purchased. Colour, style and heel height may compete equally. People, particularly women, seem to be tolerant of minor foot discomfort and it is necessary to explain that ill-fitting footwear may damage feet and that comfort should be paramount when choice of footwear is concerned.

### Length

Correctly-fitting shoes should have a gap between the longest toe and the front of the shoe to allow for elongation of the foot, which takes place when walking. This gap should ideally be about 12 mm. Shoes that are too short will be recognisable, as the upper will tend to bulge at heel and toe. There are a number of simple tests with which this observation can be confirmed. They are not all suitable for all types of shoes.

- With the patient standing in her shoes, palpate the end of the longest toe through the toe puff. This may not be possible if the toe puff is reinforced.
- Sprinkle a little talcum powder into the shoe and ask the patient to walk a few paces. When the shoes are removed an outline of the toes can be seen printed in the powder on the insole from which the gap can be assessed. It may be difficult to see the result of this test in footwear which extends high up the instep (high-waisted).
- Cut a thin strip of card the length of the foot and slide this into the shoe until it touches the tip. This should reveal a gap of about 12 mm between the inside of the heel and the end of the strip of card (Fig. 10.9). This method can be influenced by the shape of the toe puff and is therefore most effective in round-toed shoes. To minimise the error, keep the width of the card narrow and do not slide it right to the end of very pointed-toed shoes.

Shoes that are too short will mould the toes into the shape of the front of the shoe; shoes that are pointed are likely to cause pressure lesions on the toes.

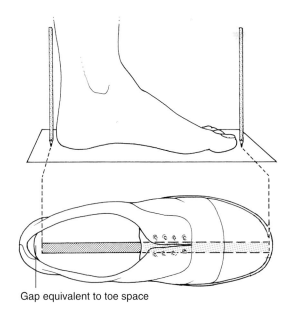

Gap equivalent to toe space

**Figure 10.9** A method of testing a shoe for correct length.

**Length of children's shoes.** Children's shoes need a little more toe space than adults to allow for growth. A gap of 20 mm between the longest toe and the front of the shoe should be present in new shoes, allowing 8–9 mm for growth before new shoes are needed. If a child's shoe is worn out it is likely that it is too small, as it is usual for young feet to outgrow the shoe before it is worn out. It is also important to check for sock fit with growing feet as these too can be rapidly outgrown. Hosiery that is too small can cause as much damage as shoes that are too short.

### Heel to ball length

Correctly-fitting heel to ball length will ensure that the hinge of the shoe is correctly aligned with the ball of the foot, and that the widest part of the foot is in the widest part of the shoe. It varies according to the design of the last. Average heel to ball length will be adequate for average feet, and will only need to be assessed if the toes are unusually short or long in relation to the rest of the foot. Heel to ball length will be incorrect if too much room for growth is allowed in children's shoes, when odd-sized feet are not fitted with different-sized shoes or when extra long shoes are bought to fit wide feet. This important measurement should only be assessed once the length of the shoes has been checked and found to be correct. Two techniques for measuring heel to ball length – one simple and one more accurate – are described below:

- With the patient standing in her shoes, feel for the metatarsophalangeal joint. If the bulge of the joint is level with the bulge of the shoe, this measurement is correct.
- Measure the distance from the patient's heel to both the first and fifth metatarsal heads. Flex the ball of the shoe and measure the distance from the heel to the point at which the shoe bends both medially and laterally. The medial and lateral measurements from the foot and the shoe should correspond.

Shoes with a heel to ball length that is too long will put unnecessary pressure and strain on the metatarsophalangeal joints, particularly that of the hallux, as the foot will be trying to flex the shoe where it is still reinforced by the shank. If the heel to ball length is too short, it will cause fewer mechanical problems but will restrict toe room (Fig. 10.10).

### Width

Correct width is also important and should be sufficient to allow the toes to rest flat on the insole without being compressed. Very few fashion shoes are made in width fittings so fashion shoes are often bought either too narrow or a size longer than they should be, to benefit from the corresponding increase in width. In a

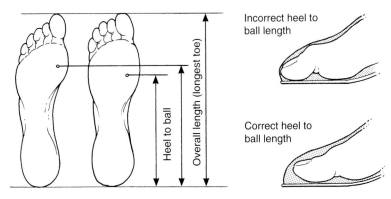

**Figure 10.10** Illustration of two feet with identical length but different heel to ball length and the result of fitting them both in the same shoe.

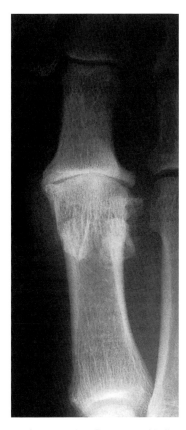

**Figure 11.27**  Osteoarthritis. This case of hallux rigidus shows complete loss of articular cartilage and early osteophytic changes at the joint periphery. There is no deviation in the joint in this case.

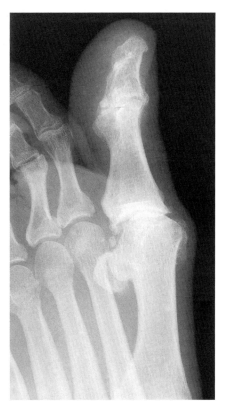

**Figure 11.28**  Osteoarthritis. This oblique view, a more advanced case than that shown in Figure 11.27, shows severe degeneration of the joint margins with obliteration of the joint space. There are multiple osteophytes, some of which have fractured away to become loose bodies within the joint capsule.

tarsal and rearfoot involvement in long-standing cases. Radiographic signs of severe pronation may often be seen.

In juvenile disorders such as Still's disease there may be retardation of long bone growth and premature epiphyseal closure, with 'spindling' of the digits.

## Osteochondrosis

This is avascular necrosis of the epiphysis or apophysis, in which there is a well-documented cycle of interference with the vascular supply to an epiphysis, possibly trauma-related but sometimes associated with endocrine dysfunction, followed by degeneration and later regeneration. It occurs in several sites on the foot, as well as in

the femoral epiphysis (*Legg–Calvé–Perthes disease*), vertebral epiphysis (*Scheuermann's disease*) and the tibial tubercle (*Osgood–Schlatter's disease*). Over 40 potential sites have been identified. In all the conditions there is a transient increase in sclerosis caused by the failure of the blood supply to remove calcium salts, followed by osteoporosis, crumbling and degeneration of the epiphysis. Revascularisation slowly occurs over a period of months and the epiphysis remodels, sometimes with residual deformity. The conditions are self-limiting and the clinical importance relates to the functional importance of the joint involved. In the foot the common conditions are as follows.

**Freiberg's infraction.** This condition affects the lesser metatarsal heads, usually the second or

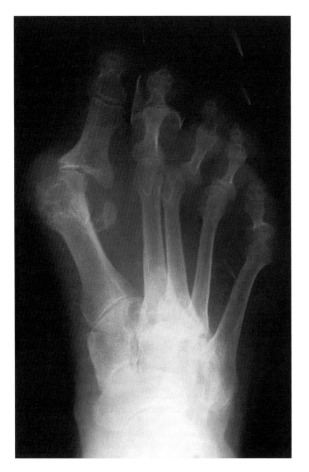

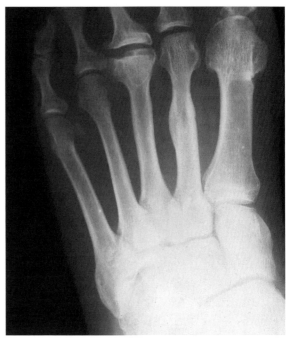

**Figure 11.30** Freiberg's infraction. The evident flattening and collapse of the third metatarsal head in this middle-aged patient is probably indicative of an old Freiberg's infraction, although this case is unconfirmed. This X-ray also shows a Keller's arthroplasty, with several loose bodies remaining around the site; an old fracture of the second metatarsal shaft; two sesamoids under the fifth metatarsal head; and a lateral exostectomy of the fifth metatarsal head.

**Figure 11.29** Rheumatoid arthritis. In this long-standing rheumatoid patient one may see gross derangement of all metatarsophalangeal joints, with subluxation in particular of the hallux and third and fourth toes. There is generalised osteoporosis and there are subchondral erosions, particularly seen around the first metatarsophalangeal joint. The midtarsal joints are also affected, with loss of bone density and joint demarcation.

third, at the age of about 12–14 years. An increase in the joint space may be noted due to the 'eggshell crush' degeneration that occurs in the metatarsal head. The finally remodelled head may be flattened or saucer-shaped. In later life it may produce secondary hypertrophic osteoarthritic degeneration (Fig. 11.30).

**Sever's disease.** Sever's disease of the calcaneal apophysis usually occurs in the age range 8–12 years. An irregularity and sclerosis may be exhibited along the apophyseal line on the poste-

rior aspect of the calcaneum. However, it should be noted that the apophyseal line is frequently irregular in any case. Some authorities believe that a diagnosis of Sever's disease cannot be made with any certainty on radiographic evidence alone.

**Köhler's disease.** Köhler's disease of the navicular occurs in youngsters in the age range 2–10 years, with a mean of 3–5 years: 70% of cases are male and there is a familial incidence. The navicular becomes dense initially, followed by porosis and collapse into a disc shape, clearly seen on a lateral view. If untreated, the bone may not regain proper form and may remain a lifelong problem.

**Other rarer conditions.** These are Iselin's disease of the fifth metatarsal base and Buschke's disease of the cuneiforms.

**Table 12.1**  Practical observational gait analysis

- Observe for amounts and timing of events
- Look for asymmetry
- Concentrate on one aspect at a time
- Bisection of calcaneus and posterior aspect of leg is often helpful
- A mark on the medial side of the navicular is also helpful
- Be aware that many individuals may consciously or subconsciously alter gait while being observed
- At least an 8–10 metre walkway is desirable with provision for watching subjects from behind/in front (frontal plane) as well as from the side (sagittal plane)
- Patient should be wearing shorts
- Observe with and without shoes and with and without orthoses

*Frontal plane observations:*
  Upper body:
      Head/eyes level or tilted?
      Shoulders level?
      Height of finger tips
      Symmetrical arm swing
      Pelvis level or tilted?
  Lower limb:
      Position of knee
      Q angle/patellar position
      Timing of knee motion
      Position of tibia
      Timing of tibial rotation
  Foot:
      Timing/amount of rearfoot motion
      Timing/amount of heel contact/off
      Timing/amount of midfoot motion
      Transfer from low gear to high gear during propulsion
      Angle and base of gait
      Abductory twist?
      Prominent extensor tendons (extensor substitution)
      Clawing of digits (flexor stabilisation)

*Sagittal plane observations*:
  Upper body:
      Forward or backward tilt
      Symmetrical arm swing
  Lower limb:
      Position/timing of hip joint motion
      Position/timing of knee joint motion
      Position/timing of ankle joint motion
  Foot:
      Timing/amount of heel lift
      Timing/amount of midtarsal joint motion
      Timing/amount of first metatarsophalangeal joint motion

There is a tendency in clinical practice to focus on frontal plane motion during the gait analysis when motion in the transverse and sagittal planes are just as important to appreciate gait. This primarily occurs for several reasons. Most clinics only have long corridors available which facilitate the observation in the frontal plane but hinders sagittal plane observation. The traditional teaching of clinical biomechanics places great importance on frontal plane compensation for different pathomechanical entities, which encourages the use of observation of gait to observe frontal plane motion of the posterior aspect of the calcaneus. The observation of the calcaneus in the frontal plane is easy, but is not necessarily indicative of any abnormal or compensatory gait patterns. For example, any abnormal compensatory movement of the calcaneus in the frontal plane is entirely dependent on the range of motion of the joints of the rearfoot complex and the orientation of the assumed position of the subtalar joint axis. If the axis is more vertical than the assumed normal, there will be very little motion of the calcaneus in the frontal plane, with more in the transverse plane. If the axis is more horizontal, there will be more motion in the frontal plane, which may not be pathological. Observational gait analysis is also limited by the ability to observe transverse plane motions and the difficulty to observe and interpret motion in all three planes simultaneously as well as motion occurring simultaneously at several joints.

In a clinical setting in patients with pathology, the observation of gait requires them to walk for some time, which can be fatiguing for them. The endurance of the patient needs to be considered.

There is no permanent record from observational gait analysis – no opportunity to review the data at a later date. The analysis is very dependent upon the skill and experience of the observer. All the data are subjective and qualitative. When one observes an individual standing on both feet, it is impossible to predict whether the load (distribution of force) under both feet is equal. This highlights the fundamental drawback of observation of gait: you cannot observe forces and the eye can be easily deceived. Reliability studies on observational gait analysis show it to be somewhat unreliable (Goodkin & Diller 1973, Krebs et al 1985, Saleh & Murdoch 1985). Despite these limitations observational gait analysis provides a good overall impression of gait and requires no equipment. Experienced observers use observational gait analysis to make critical judgements, assist in diagnosis and determine the outcomes of interventions such as foot orthoses.

**Treadmill.** One of the most debated areas of gait analysis relates to the length of walkway required in order to achieve 'normal' walking patterns: 4–6 metres is considered appropriate. Many practitioners have heightened the debate by using treadmills rather than long walkways. If a treadmill is used, one must ensure that the subject has every opportunity to adapt to treadmill walking prior to analysis being undertaken. This usually requires at least 15 minutes of walking on the treadmill. The more exposure to treadmills, the shorter the time recorded to acclimatise and perform consistently (Tollafield 1990). Clearly, older patients and those with medical conditions are likely to fatigue more quickly. No matter how sophisticated the system is, subjects must feel relaxed and comfortable when being observed. Most authorities now accept that in order to achieve this objective, the subject should be allowed to walk at his/her own cadence rather than being artificially constrained by walking in time to a metronome or some other timing device. A forced gait is of no value to a practitioner attempting to assess walking patterns.

For visual observation, treadmills facilitate closer inspection of the gait as well as easy observation of gait in the sagittal plane. Additionally, treadmills are relatively inexpensive. However, safety and balance of patients need to be paramount in their use. There are subtle differences between overground and treadmill gait that need to be taken into consideration, especially during the propulsive phase, as on the treadmill the 'ground' is moving.

**Video.** Videotaping of a movement for analysis (overground or on a treadmill) is an improvement on the traditional gait analysis. Observational gait analysis is limited by the speed that motions happen at, meaning that the more subtle motions cannot be observed in real time. Many movements take place in a very short time period. It has been observed that events that happen faster than 83 ms (1/12 second) cannot be perceived by the human eye (Gage & Ounpuu 1989), so the use of slow-motion video and freeze-frame can enhance observational gait analysis. With good pause and slow-motion facilities the finer and subtle features of gait that would otherwise be missed can be observed. This will be dependent on the frequency of sampling: below 30 Hz would be unsuitable, 50 Hz is the minimum for slow walking and 100 Hz would be required for running, or too much movement happens between each sampling frame to make the information of any use.

If two cameras and a video mixer are used, it is possible to view gait in two body planes simultaneously on the same split screen eliminating the problem of cross-plane interpretation. Initially, many practitioners do find the two views confusing. Videotapes can be archived for subsequent viewing and the comparison of before and after gaits following an intervention. Recent advances in computing now allow the taping of gait (either the traditional videotape or digital) to be viewed on a computer. Some systems (e.g. Trim-Fit™) allow the drawing and calculation of angles between segments, the generation of gait analysis reports and the linking of the recorded gait into the patient's computerised records.

Disadvantages to the use of videotaping gait are that the rotational deviations in the transverse plane cannot be seen. Movements out of the plane of the camera can also distort joint angle and influence interpretations: e.g. if sagittal plane knee motion is being observed, the angle may appear less than it really is due to internal rotation of the limb. The analysis of the videotape is still qualitative and has been shown to be only moderately reliable (Eastlock et al 1991, Keenan & Bach 1996), but it is an improvement on the straight visual observation of gait.

## METHODS OF QUANTITATIVE GAIT ANALYSIS

### Temporal and spatial parameters

As gait is repetitive, the measurement of the temporal (time) and spatial (distance) parameters are an aid to evaluating critical events that occur

# 13

# Laboratory tests

*A. Percivall*
*I. Reilly*

## INTRODUCTION

This chapter provides an overview of laboratory tests which can be performed on tissue and fluid samples from the lower limb. The tests of most relevance are:

- microbiology
- urinalysis
- blood analysis – haematology, biochemistry and serology
- histology.

The tests play a vital role in enabling the practitioner to understand the nature of local and systemic related pathologies affecting the lower limb. Data from the tests can be used to:

- provide information to aid the diagnostic process
- enable a definitive diagnosis to be made in situations where there may be a number of possible diagnoses
- measure the disease process in relation to normal parameters
- reveal occult disease processes that might affect therapeutic and treatment options
- enable implementation of effective treatment.

The accuracy of any laboratory test is determined by its sensitivity, specificity, predictive value and efficiency (see Ch. 2). Sensitivity indicates how often a positive test result is obtained from a patient with a particular disease, whereas specificity indicates the number of negative results from patients without a particular disease. Predictive values of positive test results give a measure of the frequency of the disease amongst all patients who test positive for that disease. The efficiency of a test indicates the percentage of patients correctly diagnosed with a particular pathology.

Some of the tests can be undertaken in the clinic (near patient testing) but most require the use of laboratory services. Because of the expense and possible inconvenience caused by some of the tests it is important that they are only used where appropriate.

## MICROBIOLOGY

### Indications for microbiology

Practitioners often request microbiological analysis to determine which particular organism is causing an obvious infection. However, the process can often be wasteful of both time and resources. Organisms found and identified in the laboratory usually fall into two categories: they either reflect the normal microbial flora or they fall outside this group and may be considered pathogens. It must be remembered that some normally resident organisms have the propensity to cause disease when found in abnormal sites. Conversely, just because a normal resident organism has been isolated at an abnormal site, it may not be the causative agent of the disease as commensals often contaminate samples sent to the laboratory. Further, the distinction between a pathogenic organism and a non-pathogen is often imprecise, e.g. where a person is a 'carrier' of a disease. This has led to the adoption of two basic rules:

- Never without good reason dismiss a microbe as a contaminant because it is not an 'accepted' pathogen.
- Never without good reason accept a microbe as the *necessary* cause of a disease merely because it is an 'accepted' pathogen.

Microorganisms are classified, biologically, into four main groups: viruses, protozoa, bacteria and fungi. In podiatry, with the exception of some superficial mycoses, most infections are caused by bacteria. Some viral infections of the foot do occur: the main protagonist is the human papilloma virus (HPV), which gives rise to plantar warts or verrucae.

As with other forms of laboratory testing, microbiological testing should only be considered when it is likely to serve a useful purpose. The circumstances where it is applicable are:

- when the results of testing are likely to influence the choice of treatment and result in more effective treatment for the patient
- if the results will help identify sources of infection that need to be traced.

## Sampling techniques

### Specimen types

Specimens may be divided into two groups: those from normally sterile sites and those containing a normal resident flora. The differentiation is important since samples taken from normally sterile sites need to be inoculated into enrichment media. The media provides nutrients that will allow rapid growth (or amplification) of the organisms so that enough will be available for identification. Specimens taken from sites which have resident flora will, in contrast, need to be inoculated into media containing selective agents which will suppress the growth of any commensal organisms that might mask a potential pathogen.

Ideally, when microbiological information is needed, an appropriate specimen is taken from the correct site. The specimen is transported immediately to the laboratory where it is processed quickly using the best tests, which are then correctly reported; these results are returned to the originator where they can be properly interpreted at a time when the information is relevant. Thus, it is important that the results of the work done in the laboratory are a true reflection of that specimen. Reasons for failure to report an organism originally present in a specimen include:

- a delay in examination
- the amount of specimen examined is insufficient

is used. The punch is pushed through epithelial tissue and a small section of epithelial and/or connective tissue is removed. A trephine is a similar instrument to a punch, but much more sturdy. It is used for punching holes in bone. In these cases a larger access hole is necessary. Bone samples should, wherever possible, have clear radiographs attached to assist the determination of the general appearance of the lesion. The advantage of punch biopsy lies in the small area of tissue removed. Normal tissue is not usually included. The depth of tissue sampling will depend upon the pressure applied. Punch biopsy is likely to be used where large areas have been affected and treatment cannot be undertaken at the same time. Unlike excisional biopsy it is purely a diagnostic procedure. When skin biopsy is performed it is essential to create an unobtrusive scar. In the foot, tissue around digits may require a section of bone to be removed in order to achieve closure. A surgeon specialising in feet should be consulted to reduce the risk of ischaemia.

**Needle.** Aspiration is the technique used to withdraw fluids from the body, e.g. synovial fluid. Examination of synovial fluid can be very useful when examining for the presence of uric acid crystals (gout), infection or bleeding into a joint space. Where uric acid crystals are suspected the sample of synovial fluid should be placed in absolute alcohol or placed directly on to a slide. Bursae can be aspirated. This usually leads to a temporary relief of symptoms.

### Resected organs

**Partial.** Partial resection or excisional biopsy involves the removal of all the abnormal tissue plus a section of the surrounding normal tissue. This procedure permits examination of the abnormal tissue as well as, hopefully, providing treatment at the same time. It is a surgical technique which requires high standards of asepsis. A scalpel is used to incise and then dissect the abnormal tissue and some surrounding normal tissue from the site. Haemostasis should be carefully performed to prevent unnecessary complications. Tissue from skin down to muscle, ligaments and tendon will require careful repair. Ganglion formation must be removed in total as it has a high recurrence rate. The gelatinous mass is difficult to retrieve. The thin translucent membrane should be included wherever possible. Thicker membranes suggest that they have undergone longer periods of deep trauma.

**Complete.** Whole parts, such as amputated feet, toes and excised rays, can be sent to the pathology department. Analysis of whole anatomy takes a good deal longer due to the time required to separate and fixate tissues. Bone needs to undergo a decalcification process.

## Transportation and storage

Laboratory personnel will discuss the best mode of collection to ensure that an appropriate sample for testing is achieved. Specimens labelled urgent are unwelcome unless requested during surgery where a quick result is necessary, e.g. in the case of a suspected malignancy, so that appropriate treatment can be performed concomitantly. Even small samples will take 24 hours to fix before the tissue can be usefully analysed.

All specimens should be clearly marked with the patient's name, hospital number, site and the date/time that the sample was taken. A full history of the patient is essential. High-risk cases should be identified with a separate 'high risk' label. The specimen should be sealed in a plastic bag, the request form remaining outside.

As with microbiological samples, damage can be sustained by using an incorrect method of transportation. Most tissue samples are placed in a screw-cap container containing normal buffered formalin (NBF) solution. Formalin itself constitutes a hazard, especially if spilt on living tissue. Samples for frozen section should be transported dry. They will be damaged if they come into contact with formalin. Frozen sectioning provides rapid results, usually within 5–10 minutes, and is used where results are urgently required: often when the patient is still on the operating table, when the result of the test will decide the course of action to be taken.

## Tests and interpretation of results

These fall into several categories depending upon the nature of the lesion and/or suspected pathology. Slides of tissue are produced for microscopy. Often, staining techniques are used in order to show up changes more distinctively.

The main purpose of histological examination is to assess whether the tissue or fluid sample differs from what is normal. Abnormal cellular findings, e.g. changes to the nucleus, may indicate malignant changes. Chronic inflammation may be evident because of the presence of lymphocytes, plasma cells and macrophages. Abnormal findings may relate to the presence of giant cells, a characteristic feature produced by foreign bodies. This is a common feature in the foot.

Scarring and inflammatory changes may tether down tissue, which can account for some pain syndromes in both fore and hind parts of the foot. These syndromes are difficult to diagnose accurately other than by exploratory procedures.

Nerves fall under this category. They can show marked changes, involving abnormal blood vessels, as in the case of neuromata. Nerve conduction tests may provide evidence of damage prior to surgical investigation in the foot.

## SUMMARY

This chapter has covered the indications for the use of a range of near-patient and laboratory-based tests, appropriate sampling techniques, the principles of testing and interpretation of results. Emphasis has been placed on starting with the simplest tests prior to using more specific and sophisticated tests.

The use of laboratory tests can never replace good interview and assessment techniques. Tests should be used economically and wisely, should cause no harm to the patient and above all should be used to support treatment, confirm diagnosis or rule out a suspected malignancy. Results should be acted upon in order to ensure that effective treatment is provided.

FURTHER READING

Axford J 1996 Medicine. Blackwell Science, Oxford
Bayer Diagnostics Urinalysis – the inside information
Blandy J 1998 Lecture notes on urology, 5th edn. Blackwell Science, Oxford
Hanno P M, Wein A J 1994 Clinical manual of urology. McGraw-Hill, New York
Hoffbrand A V, Pettit J E 1993 Essential haematology. Blackwell Scientific, Oxford
Karlowicz K A 1995 Urological nursing – principles and practice. W B Saunders, Philadelphia
Kumar P, Clark M 1998 Clinical medicine, 4th edn. W B Saunders, Philadelphia

Philpott-Howard J 1996 Microbiology. In: Hooper J, McCreanor G, Marshall W, Myers P (eds) Primary care and laboratory medicine. ACB Venture Publications, London
Quinn G 1995 Laboratory blood tests in podiatry. British Journal of Podiatric Medicine and Surgery 7(2): 24–27
Robinson S H, Reich P R 1993 Haematology, 3rd edn. Little, Brown and Company, Boston
Stokes E J, Ridgeway G L, Wren M W D 1993 Clinical microbiology, 7th edn. Edward Arnold, UK
Tortora G J, Grabowski S R 2000 Principles of anatomy and physiology, 9th edn. John Wiley and Sons, New York

# Specific client groups

PART CONTENTS

11.6% of their patients required treatment, whereas Rushforth (1978), in an 11-year follow-up of 83 children, found that 86% demonstrated complete resolution of the deformity.

Metatarsus adductus represents a spectrum of mild to severe deformity. Assessment of the foot's flexibility is the practitioner's primary objective (Fig. 14.10). If the foot can easily be corrected and the adductus position is mild, the prognosis for spontaneous resolution is excellent. As the deformity becomes more marked there is often a corresponding increase in rigidity. Clinical features of calcaneal eversion, medial talonavicular joint bulging and 'humping' of the dorsolateral midfoot indicate that spontaneous correction is unlikely.

Uncompensated metatarsus adductus presents as a high-arched supinated foot; symptoms are usually minimal and may be limited to skin lesions under the fifth metatarsophalangeal joint. Accordingly, prognosis is less favourable and treatment should be instigated as soon as possible. Another significant finding on assessment is the presence of a vertical crease overlying the medial cuneiform. The vertical cuneiform crease presents only in the more severely affected feet.

Radiographic examination can assist the evaluation of metatarsus adductus in cases of skew- or Z foot where rearfoot involvement exists. This complex variant of metatarsus adductus presents an everted rearfoot with plantarflexed and adducted talus. Several charting techniques have been developed to measure metatarsus adductus and its variants (Berg 1986). The value of radiography is limited. This is because the tarsal bones do not ossify until the patient is 3–4 years old; furthermore, in a non-weightbearing patient the plate will simply show the position the foot was held in for X-ray.

In metatarsus adductus parents are often concerned about the child's adducted style of gait rather than the foot shape. To ensure consistent and reliable diagnosis, all other causes of adducted gait, including internal femoral rotation, internal tibial torsion, genicular position, compensation for a forefoot valgus and hallux varus (Jimenez 1992), must be ruled out. In conclusion, the 'level of deformity' may be quite

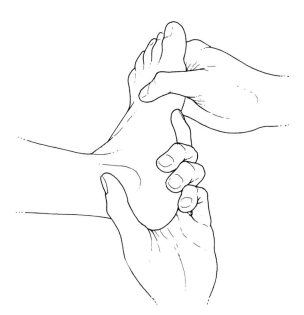

**Figure 14.10**  Assessing flexibility of the metatarsus adductus foot by cupping the heel in inversion while pushing the forefoot straight.

different. It is important therefore to note any element of these conditions which may be superimposed upon the metatarsus adductus, as management of more than one condition may be necessary.

## Congenital talipes equinovarus (clubfoot)

In congenital talipes equinovarus (CTEV), the adductus of the forefoot occurs at the midtarsal joint and not at the tarsometatarsal joint. There are four components to the deformity: equinus, inversion of the rearfoot, adductus and pronation of the forefoot. The most severe deformities, however, occur in the rearfoot. The talus is abducted and the calcaneus is in equinus. The calcaneus is also inverted, whereas the navicular is displaced medial to the head of the talus. The posterior and medial soft tissues, including tibialis posterior, flexor digitorum longus and triceps surae, are also shortened and atrophied, forming a 'pipe stem' shape to the leg.

CTEV is difficult to correct and there is a high incidence of recurrence. It is well documented

**Table 14.3** Limp relating to specific location

| Location | Possible causes |
| --- | --- |
| Nervous system CNS | Cerebral tumour<br>Cerebral palsy<br>Spina bifida<br>Spinal muscular atrophy |
| PNS/ muscle | Poliomyelitis<br>Friedreich's ataxia<br>Muscular dystrophy<br>Charcot–Marie–Tooth disease |
| Back | Trauma<br>Acute appendicitis<br>Herniated nucleus pulposus (slipped disc)<br>Scheuermann's disease of the spine (osteochondritis of spine)<br>Spondylolisthesis (forward displacement of vertebra on one distal to it) |
| Hip | Developmental dislocation of the hip (DDH)<br>Slipped capital femoral epiphysis (SCFE)<br>Transient synovitis of the hip<br>Legg–Calvé–Perthes disease<br>Trauma<br>Coxa vara (provokes waddling gait)<br>Trochanteric bursitis |
| Femur/tibia | Fracture (fractured femur may present as hip or knee pain)<br>Blount's disease<br>Limb-length inequality (short femur or tibia) |
| Knee | Osgood–Schlatter's disease (traction apophysitis)<br>Osteochondritis dissecans<br>Chondromalacia<br>Haemophilia<br>Sickle-cell anaemia<br>Rickets<br>Baker's cyst<br>Referred pain from hip |
| Ankle/foot | Fracture/sprain<br>Rickets (ankle)<br>Osteomyelitis (calcaneus)<br>Unicameral bone cyst (calcaneus)<br>Sever's disease (traction apophysitis)<br>Osteochondroses – Mouchet's or Diaz/Köhler's/ Buschke's/Freiberg's/Treve's disease<br>Haglund's disease (osteochondrosis of accessory navicular)<br>Iselin's disease (traction apophysitis)<br>Accessory navicular – type II (Romanowski & Barrington 1991)<br>Tarsal coalition<br>Embedded foreign body in foot<br>Verruca<br>Onychocryptosis<br>Subungual exostosis |
| Miscellaneous | Septic arthritis (juvenile idiopathic arthritis)<br>Angioleiomyoma<br>Leukaemia<br>Attention-seeking device<br>Child abuse |

# SUMMARY

Although the assessment process is similar, the skills required to assess the child do differ from those used to assess an adult.

Assessment of the child requires sufficient knowledge of normal development and the ability to differentiate between self-limiting developmental conditions and significant, persistent abnormalities, and those that warrant further evaluation. The practitioner must appreciate normal developmental milestones in order to undertake a thorough assessment.

This chapter has primarily concentrated on common paediatric orthopaedic conditions of the lower limb. Brief discussion has considered pertinent vascular, dermatological and arthritic conditions that lead to patients seeking advice. The practitioner must identify the cause of any pain and be vigilant for signs of neuromuscular deficit. In a well-resourced nation such as the UK, most severe problems associated with the foot and lower limb are detected at birth. However, all practitioners should be aware of problems that may have missed detection or which are relatively mild but may still lead to functional problems in later life.

## REFERENCES

Alvik L 1960 Increased anteversion of the femoral neck as a sole sign of dysplasia coxae. Acta Orthopaedica Scandinavica 29: 301–306

Apgar V 1953 Evaluation of the newborn infant. Current Research Anesthesia Analgesics 32: 260

Beeson P 1988 Juvenile chronic arthritis: the foot. The Chiropodist 43(2): 20–26

Beeson P 1990 The clinical significance for chiropodists of recent advances made in the pathology and treatment of psoriasis. Journal British Podiatric Medicine 45(3): 43–46

Beeson P 1995 Podiatric perspective: a case study of rheumatoid arthritis and a multidisciplinary approach. British Journal Therapy Rehabilitation 2(10): 566–571

Beeson P 1999 Frontal plane configuration of the knee in children. The Foot 9(1): 18–26

Beighton P H, Grahame R, Bird H A 1989 Hypermobility of joints, 2nd edn. Springer, Berlin

Berg E E 1986 A reappraisal of metatarsus adductus and skewfoot. Journal Bone and Joint Surgery [Am] 68-A: 1185–1196

Blane W A, Mattison D R, Kane R 1971 LDS intrauterine amputations and amniotic band syndrome. Lancet 2: 158

Bulbena A, Duro J C, Porta M et al 1992 Clinical assessment of hypermobility of joints: assembling criteria. Journal Rheumatology 19(1): 115–122

Cahuzac J Ph, Vardon D, Sales de Gauzy J 1995 Development of the clinical tibiofemoral angle in normal adolescents. Journal Bone and Joint Surgery [Br] 77-B: 729–732

Coleman S S 1994 Developmental dislocation of the hip: evolutionary changes in diagnosis and treatment [Editorial]. Journal Pediatric Orthopedics 14: 1–2

Davids J R 1996 Pediatric knee: clinical assessment and common disorders. Pediatric Clinics of North America 43(5): 1067–1090

DeValentine S D 1992 Foot and ankle disorders in children. Churchill Livingstone, New York, pp 452–458

Elftman H 1945 Torsion of the lower extremity. American Journal Physiology and Anthropology 3: 255–265

Fabry G, McEwan G D, Shands A R 1973 Torsion of the femur (a follow up study in normal and abnormal conditions). Journal Bone and Joint Surgery [Am] 55A: 1726–1738

Fields L 1981 The limping child: a review of the literature. Journal American Podiatric Association 71(2): 60–64

Gauthier G, Elbaz R 1979 Freiberg's infraction: a subchondral bone fatigue fracture. A new surgical treatment. Clinical Orthopedics Related Research 142: 93–95

Giladi M, Milgrom C, Stein M et al 1985 The low arch, a protective factor in stress fractures. Orthopedic Review 14: 709–712

Harris E J 1997 Hip instability encountered in pediatric podiatry practice. Clinics in Podiatric Medicine and Surgery 14(1): 179–208

Harris R I 1965 Peroneal spastic flat foot (rigid valgus foot). Journal Bone and Joint Surgery [Am] 47-A: 1657–1667

Harris M-C R, Beeson P 1988a Is there a link netween juvenile hallux abducto valgus and generalised hypermobility ? A review of the literature. Part I. The Foot 8(3): 125–128

Harris M-C R, Beeson P 1988b Generalised hypermobility: is it a predisposing factor towards the development of juvenile hallux abducto valgus ? Part 2. The Foot 8(4): 203–209

Heath C H, Staheli L T 1993 Normal limits of knee angle in white children – genu varum and genu valgum. Journal Pediatric Orthopedics 13: 259–262

Hensinger R N 1986 Limp. Pediatric Clinics of North America 33(6): 1355–1364

Hubbard D D, Staheli L T, Chew D E 1988 Medial femoral torsion and osteoarthrosis. Journal Pediatric Orthopedics 8: 540–542

Hutter C G, Scott W 1949 Tibial torsion. Journal Bone and Joint Surgery [Am] 31-A: 511–518

Jiminez A L 1992 Hallux varus. In: McGlamry D E, Banks A S, Downey M S (eds) Comprehensive textbook of foot surgery, 2nd edn. Williams & Wilkins, Baltimore, pp 587–588

Johnston O 1959 Further studies of the inheritance of hand and foot anomalies. Clinical Orthopedics 8: 146–159

Katz K, Rosenthal A, Yosipovitch Z 1992 Normal ranges of popliteal angle in children. Journal Pediatric Orthopedics 12: 229–231

Kilmartin T E 1988 Medial genicular rotation: aetiology and management. The Chiropodist 43: 181–184

Kilmartin T E, Barrington R L, Wallace W A 1991 Metatarsus primus varus. Journal Bone and Joint Surgery [Br] 73B: 937–940

Kilmartin T E, Barrington R L, Wallace W A 1994 A controlled prospective trial of a foot orthosis in the treatment of juvenile hallux valgus. Journal Bone and Joint Surgery [Br] 76B: 210–214

Kulik S A, Clanton T O 1996 Tarsal coalition. Foot and Ankle International 17(5): 286–296

Kyne P J, Mankin H J 1965 Changes in intra-articular pressure with subtalar joint motion with special reference to the etiology of peroneal spastic flat foot. Bulletin of the Hospital for Joint Diseases 26: 181–186

Lang L M G, Volpe R G 1998 Measurement of tibial torsion. Journal American Podiatric Medical Association 88(4): 160–165

LaPorta G 1973 Torsional abnormalities. Archives Podiatric Medical Foot Surgery 1: 47–61

Luder J 1988 Early recognition of cerebral palsy. Update 15 March: 1955–1963

McRae R 1997 Clinical orthopaedic examination. Churchill Livingstone, Edinburgh, pp 231–238

Malleson P N, Southwood T R 1993 The epidemiology of arthritis: an overview. In: Southwood T R, Malleson P N (eds) Baillière's clinical paediatrics international practice and research. Baillière Tindall, London, 1: 635–636

Meadow R 1992 Difficult and unlikeable parents. Archives Disease in Childhood 67: 697–702

Michele A A, Nielsen P M 1976 Tibiotalar torsion: bioengineering paradigm. Orthopedic Clinics of North America 7: 929–947

Morley A J M 1957 Knock knees in children. British Medical Journal 2: 976–979

Mosier K M, Asher M 1984 Tarsal coalitions and peroneal spastic flat foot. Journal Bone and Joint Surgery [Am] 66-A: 976–984

Napolitano C, Walsh S, Mahoney L et al 2000 Risk factors that may adversely modify the natural history of the paediatric pronated foot. Clinics in Podiatric Medicine and Surgery 17(3): 397–417

Novacheck T F 1996 Developmental dysplasia of the hip. Pediatric Clinics of North America 43: 829–848

Ponsetti I V 1992 Current concepts review. Treatment of congenital clubfoot. Journal Bone and Joint Surgery [Am] 74-A: 448–454

Ponsetti I V 1996 Congenital clubfoot – Fundamentals of treatment. Oxford University Press, Oxford, pp 68–80

Ponsetti I V, Becker J R 1966 Congenital metatarsus adductus, the results of treatment. Journal Bone and Joint Surgery [Am] 74-A: 702–711

Reade E, Hom L, Hallum A et al 1984 Changes in popliteal angle measurement in infants up to one year of age. Developmental Medicine Child Neurology 26: 774–780

Reikeras O, Hoiseth A 1989 Torsion of the leg determined by computerised tomography. Acta Orthopaedica Scandinavica 60: 330–333

Romanowski C A J, Barrington N A 1991 The accessory ossicles of the foot. The Foot 1(2): 61–70

Rose G K, Welton E A, Marshall T 1985 The diagnosis of flat foot in the child. Journal Bone and Joint Surgery [Br] 67-B: 71–78

Rushforth G F 1978 The natural history of hooked forefoot. Journal Bone and Joint Surgery [Br] 60-B: 530–532

Salenius P, Vankka E 1975 The development of the tibio-femoral angle in children. Journal Bone and Joint Surgery [Am] 57-A: 259–261

Sharrard W J W 1976 Intoeing and flat feet. British Medical Journal 1: 888–889

Smillie I S 1969 Treatment of Freiberg's infraction. Procedures of Royal Society of Medicine 60: 29–31

Staheli L T 1993 Rotational problems in childhood. Journal Bone and Joint Surgery 75-A: 939–949

Staheli L T, Lippert F, Denotter P 1977 Femoral anteversion and physical performance in adolescent and adult life. Clinical Orthopedics 129: 213–216

Staheli L T, Chew D E, Corbett M 1987 The longitudinal arch. Journal Bone and Joint Surgery [Am] 69-A: 426–428

Svenningsen S, Tierjesen T, Auflem M 1990 Hip rotation and intoeing gait. Clinical Orthopaedics Related Research 251: 177–182

Tachdjian M O 1972 Pediatric orthopaedics, 2nd edn, Vol 4. W B Saunders, Philadelphia, p 2826

Tachdjian M O 1985 The child's foot. W B Saunders, Philadelphia

Tax H 1985 Podopaediatrics, 2nd edn. Williams & Wilkins, Baltimore, pp 90–97

Thackeray C, Beeson P 1996a In-toeing gait in children: a review of the literature. The Foot 6(1): 1–4

Thackeray C, Beeson P 1996b Is in-toeing gait a developmental stage ? The Foot 6(1): 19–24

Torpin R 1968 Fetal malformations caused by amniotic rupture during gestation. Charles C Thomas, Springfield

Turner M S, Smillie I S 1981 The effect of tibial torsion on the pathology of the knee. Journal Bone and Joint Surgery [Br] 63-B: 396–398

Valmassy R L 1993 In: Thomson P (ed) Introduction to podopaediatrics. W B Saunders, London, pp 29–31

Wallander H, Hansson G, Tjernstrom B 1996 Correction of persistent clubfoot deformities with the Ilizarov external fixator. Acta Orthopaedica Scandinavica 67(3): 283–287

Waugh W 1958 The ossification and vascularisation of the tarsal navicular and their relation to Köhler's disease. Journal Bone and Joint Surgery [Br] 403-B: 765–768

## FURTHER READING

Berkow R (ed) 1987 The Merck manual, 15th edn. Merck Sharp & Dohme Research Laboratories

Behrman R E, Vaughan V C 1987 Nelson textbook of pediatrics, 13th edn. W B Saunders, Philadelphia

Drennan J 1992 The child's foot and ankle. Ravens Press, New York

Ferrari J 1998 A review of the foot deformities seen in juvenile chronic arthritis. The Foot 8(4): 193–196

Illingworth R S 1990 The development of the infant and the young child. Churchill Livingstone, Edinburgh

McCrea J D 1985 Pediatric orthopaedics of the lower extremity. Futura, New York

Pollak M 1993 Textbook of developmental paediatrics. Churchill Livingstone, Edinburgh

Sharrard M D 1979 Paediatric orthopaedics and fractures, Vols I and II, 2nd edn. Blackwell Scientific, London

Sheridan M D 1980 From birth to five years. Children's developmental progress, 7th edn. NFER-Nelson Publishing, Berkshire

Thomson P (ed) 1993 Introduction to podopaediatrics. W B Saunders, London

assessment should include examination of the joints, muscles and osseous alignment (Ch. 8). The majority of podiatric interventions in sports injuries are related to the assessment and treatment of structural alignment and function that has caused or contributed to the injury.

Chronic or overuse sports injuries are usually due to the presence of one or both of the following situations:

- normal structure and function but inadequate preparation or excessive demands placed on the tissues
- abnormal structure and function with relatively normal demands placed on the tissues.

Although this is a rather simplistic view, it can be seen to be true in the majority of cases. If we consider two runners with patellofemoral syndrome: runner A runs over 100 miles/week, running every day; runner B runs 20 miles/week, running 3 times per week with 4 rest days. Apart from their injuries, they are both healthy and have taken 6 months to get to this weekly mileage. It should be clear that runner A is doing too much, too soon, and too frequently:

- running 100 miles/week will often result in injury
- a running volume of 100 miles/week in just 6 months has not allowed the tissues to undergo the normal adaptive processes required to meet these demands
- running every day does not allow adequate recovery time for the tissues, resulting in injury.

Other aetiological factors may also be present in runner A, but treatment will fail unless the errors of the training schedule are addressed. In the case of runner B, the aetiology of his injury is likely to be due to abnormal structure and function which has resulted in excessive patellofemoral joint reaction forces. His structural assessment should include examination of factors such as:

- muscle inflexibility (hamstrings, iliotibial band, quadriceps, lateral retinacula of the knee and calf muscles)

- muscle weakness (vastus medialis, gluteus medius, medial retinacula of the knee)
- patella malalignment or hypermobility (in frontal, transverse or sagittal plane)
- patella maltracking (during flexion and extension)
- excessive subtalar joint pronation
- frontal plane malalignment of the knee or tibia.

The presence or absence of these factors should assist the practitioner in identifying the aetiological factors and planning the most effective treatment (Witvrouw et al 2000).

Asymmetries between limbs may represent the obvious cause of a unilateral overuse injury. However, it is important to consider the role of other factors such as the type of activity, exercise surface, unilateral trauma and injury history. Any of these factors may cause a unilateral injury. If structural asymmetry is identified, then the practitioner must determine a biomechanical mechanism by which the asymmetry could have caused the overuse injury. If we consider stress fractures as an example, there is a strong association between stress fractures and limb-length inequality (Brukner et al 1999). Stress fractures tend to occur in the longer limb, and the greater the inequality the greater the incidence (Friberg 1982). The reasons for this are thought to be due to the biomechanical consequences of the limb-length difference, which results in a longer stance phase, skeletal realignment, greater osseous torsion and increased muscle activity of the longer limb.

### Flexibility

Hypermobility due to increased muscle flexibility and ligamentous laxity has been associated with a greater risk of injury. Hypermobility is often determined by the Beighton score, which is based on a nine-point test designed to measure excessive joint movement (Ch. 14). This test has been used in a number of studies on flexibility and injury, which has generally shown that hypermobility is associated with a greater incidence of ligamentous injury. Rossiter & Galbraith

(1996) found that hypermobility was present in 34% of military recruits with ankle and knee ligament injuries compared with 19% of control subjects. Increased flexibility, measured by the sit and reach test, in the absence of ligamentous laxity has not been shown to be a significant factor in injury prediction.

Generalised inflexibility due to muscle tightness has been linked to musculotendinous injury: while this is likely to be true, it has not been proven in any long-term prospective study. However, if a theoretical causal link can be made between the muscle inflexibility and the injury, then stretching of those muscles should be included in the treatment programme. Likewise, if hypermobility is present, then stretching should be avoided and athletes encouraged to perform specific stabilising exercises.

Stretching prior to activity does not appear to reduce the risk of lower limb injury. This has been demonstrated in a number of studies, including two large randomised controlled trials involving military recruits (Pope et al 1998, 2000). These studies did not measure the level of flexibility of the two groups but demonstrated that the injury incidences of the two groups were the same irrespective of whether the athlete stretched or not prior to exercise. This does not mean that injured athletes with muscle inflexibility should not be instructed to stretch, as this is an effective treatment modality. However, athletes are often questioned as to whether they stretch before and after activity and encouraged to do so if they do not. There seems little evidence to support this premise and failure to stretch before exercise should not be viewed as a risk factor to injury.

### Physical fitness

Physical fitness is known to lower the risk of injury, as shown in a number of studies based on military and civilian populations (Neely 1998). This protective mechanism not only applies to practising a known sport but also to learning a new sport or athletic skill. The level of reduced risk varies amongst the studies, and is dependent upon the activity being undertaken and the fitness test used. Pope et al (2000) were able to demonstrate that the least-fittest group of their army recruits were 14 times more likely to sustain a lower limb injury than the fittest group. The fitness method used was the progressive 20 m shuttle run test, also known as the bleep test. This test is one of the most popular fitness tests used today.

When assessing injured athletes it is important to gauge their fitness level, as you may need to offer advice on a more appropriate training regimen. This is often the case for the novice athlete who enthusiastically embarks on an over-ambitious fitness programme. This will result in injury, as the musculoskeletal system is not prepared for such strenuous exercise. When an injury occurs, the athlete should be advised to modify his exercise to prevent recurrence or further injury to other structures. This advice may include changing the method of exercise or reducing the intensity, frequency or duration of the exercise.

### Physical build

The relationship of physical strength to injury is unknown. To avoid injury the musculoskeletal system must be able to cope with the physical demand of the sporting activity. Some evidence suggests that stronger athletes are more injury prone (Knapik et al 1992). The reasons for this are unclear, but it may be that the muscular forces generated by stronger athletes damage their joint structures and even the muscles themselves. It may also be that stronger athletes exercise at greater intensity or duration than weaker athletes, resulting in higher injury rates.

There is a correlation between strength imbalance and injury that is most frequently seen in the knee joint, where differences between hamstring and quadriceps strengths have been associated with cruciate ligament injuries. The role of strength differences between limbs has also shown a greater injury incidence on the weaker side. There is general agreement that strength differences greater than 10% can increase the injury risk to the weaker limb. These injuries may be acute, as with cruciate ligament injuries, or chronic, due to fatigue, e.g. tendonitis, muscle strains and stress fractures. The role of limb dominance in injury incidence is less certain. Limb dominance in racket or ball sports is associated with different injury patterns. However, in sports that require equal stresses through both limbs there is no evidence to suggest limb dominance is a risk factor. Herring (1993) was unable to show any difference in injury incidence based on limb dominance in elite runners.

Anthropometric data such as height, weight, body mass index (BMI) and total body fat have also been examined as injury risk factors. In general, it is only the BMI that has been shown to be a positive indicator for injury risk. The BMI is determined by dividing the body weight in kilograms by the height of the patient in metres squared (i.e. $kg/m^2$). The normal BMI range is 20–25 with above 25 representing clinically overweight, above 30 clinically obese and below 20 representing underweight. As a general rule, the injury risk doubles for individuals who fall outside the normal BMI range.

### Psychological factors

Psychological factors can play a significant part in both the development of a sports injury and the rehabilitation of the injury. Although there is no definite psychological profile of the injury-prone athlete, there are certain characteristics which may predispose the athlete to injury. Acute injuries may be more frequently seen in athletes who are extroverts with a low sense of responsibility. These athletes are natural risk-takers who may put themselves in injurious situations unnecessarily. The reasons for this type of sporting behaviour may be due to a daredevil attitude, poor decision making or an attempt to gain popularity with their peers, coach or supporters.

Chronic overuse injuries may be seen more frequently in athletes who demonstrate high levels of responsibility and dedication. These athletes will often train and play beyond the point of fatigue, resulting in small repetitive trauma to the tissues. This can cause chronic overuse injuries such as stress fractures, tendonitis and muscle strains.

Other obvious psychological injury risk factors are stress and anxiety levels. Stress may come from the sport itself or other life stresses. Changes in personal circumstances, careers and relationships with family and friends can induce significant stress on an athlete. The athlete may then view sport as an escape or outlet to vent frustration, which can lead to poor decision making and injury. It is important to be aware of these factors when treating the athlete, as injury recurrence will be high if they are not addressed. This may mean liaising with the athlete's coach or team physician, so that an appropriate social support network can be provided.

The psychological response of the athlete to an injury can vary significantly. Most will go through a reaction of stress and grief. The grief response to an injury is like a minor or moderate version of losing a loved one. The severity of the injury and the importance of sport to the athlete will determine the level of the grief response. The grief response is characterised by three phases:

**Phase 1 – shock.** The immediate response to the injury may be one of sudden complete shock. The athlete may show signs of anger, disbelief and deny the existence of the injury. Rehabilitation of the athlete cannot begin until this phase is over.

**Phase 2 – preoccupation.** The athlete may demonstrate signs of depression and guilt about the injury, becoming isolated from other team members, family and friends. The athlete may also show signs of bargaining behaviour when undergoing treatment during this phase. Rehabilitation may begin during this phase, but real progress will not be achieved until the athlete enters the next phase.

**Phase 3 – reorganisation.** This is characterised by the athlete fully accepting the presence of the injury and demonstrating a renewed interest in the rehabilitation programme. The athlete is also likely to show a renewed interest in the sport and in relationships with family and team-mates.

The practitioner should be aware of the various emotional states the athlete may demonstrate. This can help in formulating more appropriate treatment plans with one of the main aims being to guide the athlete to the final reorganisation phase.

### Systemic disease

Practitioners must be aware that not all athletes are free from systemic disease or medical conditions. Cardiovascular, respiratory, endocrine, arthritic and neurological complaints are seen fairly frequently in the athletic population. The spur for many people to start to exercise may be the presence of hypertension, cardiovascular disease or obesity. Patients with systemic disease are often prescribed exercise programmes by other medical professionals such as GPs, medical consultants or physiotherapists. The role of exercise and sport is generally beneficial for patients with systemic disease as it can improve cardiovascular, respiratory and neurological function and help improve strength, flexibility and mobility. However, the exercise must be of the right type, intensity, duration and frequency to ensure medical complications do not arise. Practitioners should also be aware that undiagnosed systemic disease may be the underlying cause of the injury (Case history 15.3).

Patients with cardiovascular conditions such as peripheral vascular disease or hypertension must exercise with caution. Dynamic exercise increases the cardiac output, increases the blood flow to working muscles and causes peripheral vasodilation. The net result is a rise in systolic pressure in normotensive athletes. However, with hypertension there are rises in both systolic and diastolic pressures from already elevated baseline levels. This can elevate the blood pressure to dangerous levels, particularly if the athlete has moderate to severe hypertension, the exercise intensity is too high or isometric exercise is performed.

In patients with vasospastic conditions or peripheral vascular disease, localised tissue hypoxia can result if the metabolic demands of the exercising tissues are greater than the blood supply can provide. It is also important to remember that certain sports injuries are caused by cardiovascular changes such as acute and chronic compartment syndromes of the lower leg and foot, and popliteal artery entrapment syndrome. Exercise can also occasionally be the cause of cardiovascular pathology, such as effort-induced deep vein thrombosis or external artery endofibrosis (Bradshaw 2000).

---

Case history 15.3

A 38-year-old male physical education instructor was referred by his GP with a 2-month history of localised pain in both forefeet. The patient was otherwise healthy and participated in a wide variety of sports both at work and socially. Both he and his GP were unsure of the nature of his pain and he had been referred for further investigation and orthotic treatment if appropriate.

A thorough medical history demonstrated no major illnesses, operations or a history of lower limb injuries. There was no significant family medical history or social history. There was also no recent history of a change in exercise pattern or footwear. The pain was centred around the left fifth and right third metatarsophalangeal joints and tended to occur after activity. The pain was gradually getting worse. Moderate swelling was present at both joints, particularly in the right second interspace, with slight splaying of the second and third toes (Sullivan's sign). A list of differential diagnoses was considered, including stress fracture, capsulitis, synovitis, flexor digitorum longus tendonitis, neuroma, bursitis, soft tissue mass (right foot only), osteoarthritis

and systemic joint disease. After a thorough clinical examination osteoarthritis, stress fracture and tendonitis were excluded. The examination of the joints caused pain and there were some neuritic symptoms in the right foot. The patient was given a local anaesthetic injection into the web space to exclude a Morton's neuroma and a temporary orthosis. The patient was also referred for X-ray.

Upon review the local anaesthetic injection had not resolved the symptoms but the temporary orthosis had alleviated some of the pain. The X-rays revealed erosive changes in both metatarsal heads and the patient was subsequently diagnosed by a rheumatologist as having rheumatoid arthritis. The patient is currently taking disease-modifying drugs, wearing appropriate orthoses and continues to exercise. His exercise programme has been modified to avoid high-impact and contact sports. This case demonstrates the importance of keeping an open mind when determining the diagnosis of an injury. Practitioners should consider all potential causes to avoid unnecessary or inappropriate treatment.

Athletes with diabetes must monitor their blood glucose levels very closely, especially when starting or altering an exercise programme. Exercise increases the demand for glucose in the exercising tissues, resulting in a sharp drop in blood glucose levels. This can trigger a hypoglycaemic attack. Athletes will often have to reduce their dosage of insulin before exercise and should always have a ready source of glucose available when they exercise. It is important that diabetics exercise to help reduce cardiovascular complications and limited joint mobility associated with the disease.

Neurological conditions such as upper or lower motor neurone lesions, hereditary motor and sensory neuropathies and nerve entrapments may occur in athletes. Patients with neurological disorders are often advised to exercise. Such patients may have altered sensation, altered muscle function and gait and a pes cavus foot deformity. These patients must be carefully assessed to ensure they undertake the appropriate exercise programme using appropriate supports as required. Avoidance of high-impact and contact sports is essential in neuropathic patients.

## Extrinsic factors

### Sporting equipment

The most important piece of sporting equipment in the assessment of chronic overuse injuries is the athlete's footwear. The athlete's shoes can assist in the diagnosis of the injury as they are often a contributory aetiological factor. They also represent an adjunct to treatment, as the practitioner will often modify the footwear or use it to accommodate an orthosis. In certain circumstances the practitioner may recommend changing the footwear completely. Recommending the right shoe for the patient is not easy. Sports shoe manufacturing is a multi-billion pound industry and company research data on shoe design and function are closely guarded secrets. Each company produces a number of different models for the same sport making it hard to know which is the best one. The most expensive model does not mean it is the best. The use of 'motion control systems' or special air or gel pockets to aid shock absorption is often used to market the brand as being better than that of the competition. The evidence to support such claims is often lacking.

The practitioner should appraise the athlete's shoe, identifying good and bad attributes and, if recommending a change in footwear, advise the athlete of what to look for when buying new sports shoes. To recommend one specific model for all patients will fail, as many patients will return dissatisfied if the injury does not resolve or complain that the shoe is uncomfortable.

The aim for the practitioner is to ensure that the patient is exercising in a shoe that is:

- comfortable
- correct fit in length and width
- appropriate for the patient's sport
- does not show signs of excessive wear
- has appropriate tread, studs, spikes, cleats for the sport and exercise surface
- provides sufficient shock absorption, especially in the midsole
- provides appropriate motion control for the patient
- firm fastening
- lightweight.

Many sports shoes do not meet all of these criteria and can play a significant part in the development of an overuse injury. Worn shoes have been identified as risk factors in the incidence of a number of injuries such as stress fractures, exercise-induced leg pain and Achilles tendonitis due to a lack of shock absorption (Gardner et al 1988, Myburgh et al 1988). The shoe is the interface between the foot and the ground and must absorb significant ground reaction forces generated by sporting activity. As the shoe ages or becomes more worn, its ability to absorb these forces is reduced, resulting in increased forces being passed on to the musculoskeletal system. It has been estimated that the average running shoe loses 50% of its shock-absorbing capabilities after 300–500 miles of running (Cook et al 1985). Old shoes may not only demonstrate signs of excessive wear but also material degradation can occur, even further reducing the shock-absorbing capabilities of the shoe.

An uneven wear pattern on the sole of the shoe or the insole inside the shoe can give a guide to biomechanical abnormalities or sporting technique of the athlete. Excessive lateral wear of the rearfoot can indicate a varus alignment or strike pattern and may cause inversion ankle sprains or lateral foot and leg injuries. Excessive wear across the ball of the foot will cause a loss of traction and control, which may induce injury. Different wear patterns between the shoes may indicate different biomechanics or sporting technique. The most common example of uneven wear is limb-length inequality due to structural, functional or environmental factors.

The weight of the shoe is important to optimise performance: the heavier the shoe, the greater the muscle exertion and energy expenditure. This can cause fatigue in the lower leg muscles and therefore affect performance. Light running shoes may enhance speed but should only be worn for racing as they do not offer appropriate support or shock absorption.

The importance of comfort and correct fit cannot be overstated. Shoes that are too tight or narrow will obviously cause irritation, resulting in corns, calluses, subungual haematomas and other nail pathologies. It is common in kicking sports such as soccer and rugby that the athlete will wear a boot that is too small in order to get a better 'feel' for kicking the ball. This practice should be discouraged as it can often lead to clawing of the toes and exacerbate nail pathologies. Shoes that are too narrow or fastened too tightly can cause pain in the arch and neuritic pain in the forefoot during exercise. A shoe that is too long will allow excessive movement of the foot, resulting in friction blisters and heel slippage.

### Exercise surface

The role that the exercise surface may play in the development of overuse injuries is a contentious issue. It was previously thought that athletes who exercise on hard unyielding surfaces such as concrete would have an increased incidence of osteoarthritis due to accelerated wear and tear of the joints. There is very little evidence to support this despite several long-term prospective studies. However in athletics, harder synthetic track surfaces can increase performance but also increase the incidence of musculoskeletal injury. If athletes exercise solely on hard surfaces, increases in the incidence of medial tibial stress syndrome by 28% and Achilles tendonitis by 17% have been demonstrated (Nigg & Yeadon 1987).

Artificial grass was first used for sport in 1964 and has since become a major playing surface in a wide number of sporting activities. The injury profile of this surface is different to that of natural grass. Bowers & Martin (1976) identified an injury virtually unique to this surface. Turf toe is a hyperextension injury of the first metatarsophalangeal joint resulting in a sprain of the plantar capsuloligamentous structures. It is caused by shoes with a flexible sole in the forefoot bending excessively on a hard unyielding surface. It is primarily seen in American football but can occur in any sport played on artificial grass surfaces such as AstroTurf.

Harder surfaces invoke greater ground reaction forces, which must be absorbed by the shoe and musculoskeletal system. The body absorbs these forces primarily through the joints and eccentric muscle activity. The harder the exercise surface, the greater the eccentric muscle activity (Richie et al 1993). Theoretically, exercising on harder surfaces should cause greater knee flexion, ankle dorsiflexion and greater or prolonged subtalar joint pronation to aid the absorption of the higher ground reaction forces. No biomechanical studies have shown this to date.

In addition to the hardness of the exercise surface, it is important to consider the friction and energy loss of the surface. Friction, or horizontal stiffness, is integral in acceleration and deceleration. Artificial athletic surfaces have greater friction than grass, allowing greater acceleration and deceleration. However, these greater frictional forces must be absorbed by the body and can result in increased injuries. These injuries may be to the musculotendinous units or the ligaments designed to limit joint movements such as the cruciate ligaments of the knee.

Energy loss of a surface is related to its elastic behaviour and deformation properties. Surfaces that deform when loaded are termed compliant and result in increased contact time. This increases cushioning as peak contact forces are reduced. However, it may reduce performance as the contact time is greater, resulting in slower acceleration. Exercising on softer surfaces can also alter joint positions. Consider an athlete running on sand. The greatest contact force occurs at heel strike, so the sand will be maximally displaced at this time. This results in greater ankle dorsiflexion, requiring greater muscle activity of the calf muscles. Thus, exercising on softer surfaces may reduce injuries associated with high-impact forces but may lead to increases in muscle activity resulting in musculotendinous injury.

It is also important to consider the terrain and incline of the exercise surface. Uneven terrain such as grass will mean the body having to adapt to maintain ground contact and stability. These adaptive changes mainly occur in the frontal plane and can result in greater supinatory and pronatory moments within the foot and ankle. If these forces become excessive then frontal plane injury will result. The most obvious example of this is the inversion ankle sprain. Pronatory injuries can occur and usually involve the posterior tibial tendon. If an athlete exercises on uneven terrain with frontal plane movements of the foot and ankle limited by strapping, a brace or boots, then greater forces will be transferred to the knee. This can result in collateral ligament and cruciate damage. This injury pattern has been seen in skiing. Uneven terrain can also exist on surfaces which are perceived to be flat. The camber of roads is usually canted up to 14°. This can cause pronatory moments on one limb and supinatory moments on the other, resulting in an environmental limb-length difference.

The importance of exercising on an incline should not be overlooked. Both uphill and downhill running are associated with different joint angular relationships and muscle activity patterns. Uphill running requires greater ankle joint dorsiflexion and eccentric calf and hamstring muscle activity. Downhill running requires greater ankle plantarflexion and eccentric muscle activity of the foot dorsiflexors. This particularly affects the tibialis anterior muscle, which becomes active for longer and elongates further as it decelerates foot slap. Downhill running also increases the load on the quadriceps muscles and is known to exacerbate conditions such as patellofemoral syndrome and patella tendonitis.

### Sporting activity

The type of sport the athlete plays and the techniques they use are integral to the development of overuse injuries. Certain injuries are even named after certain sports or activities (Table 15.2). This does not mean that these injuries are unique to that particular sport, but they occur frequently due to the forces the anatomical structure has to absorb. Metatarsal stress fractures are not unique to military personnel who march, but this activity involves repetitive impact forces through the forefoot, which can result in a stress fracture. Patella tendonitis is most commonly seen in jumping sports due to the high ground reaction forces (up to eight times body weight) that this activity produces. A significant component of these forces is absorbed by eccentric quadriceps activity, which can cause patella tendonitis.

**Table 15.2** Common injuries named after a sport

| Injury name | Injury definition |
| --- | --- |
| Footballer's ankle | Anterior ankle impingement |
| Tennis leg | Rupture/tear of medial head of gastrocnemius |
| Fresher's leg | Exercise-induced shin pain |
| March fracture | Metatarsal stress fracture |
| Jumper's knee | Patella tendonitis |
| Runner's knee | Patellofemoral syndrome |
| Golfer's elbow | Medial epicondylitis |
| Tennis elbow | Medial (forehand) epicondylitis, lateral (backhand) epicondylitis |
| Swimmer's shoulder | Rotator cuff pathology |

It is important the practitioner has an understanding of the type of sport the athlete plays and its biomechanics. This will help the practitioner:

- understand the forces involved in the sport
- identify the structures at risk of injury
- determine the potential biomechanical mechanism of injury
- formulate the most appropriate treatment plan.

These four factors are all interrelated. Identifying the structures most at risk of injury requires knowledge of the forces involved in the sport. This knowledge is related to the biomechanical movements of that particular sport. Determining the biomechanical mechanism of injury is crucial to formulating the most appropriate treatment plan.

Without this knowledge it is difficult to reduce or prevent the forces that caused the injury. Appropriate treatment planning must also take into account the limitations of the sport on the treatment. This will include the athletes' footwear and other sporting equipment. Some sports do not allow the use of mechanical supports as they may compromise player safety or give the athlete an unfair advantage.

It is also important to be aware of individual variation in sporting technique, which not only determines the athlete's skill and ability at a sport but can also predispose injury. Minor differences in sporting technique can have a significant effect on injury development. An example is in running techniques between forefoot and rearfoot strikers. Forefoot striking is associated with increased impact forces, a reduced stance phase and reduced subtalar joint pronation. These three factors combined could increase the forces being absorbed both in the forefoot and more proximally in the calf muscles, shin and knee.

The team position will also help determine the sporting technique of the athlete. The position played may be based on anthropometric characteristics, limb dominance and skill levels. Team position may be important to the practitioner, as the biomechanical movements and sporting techniques used by the athlete can vary.

This will result in different injury profiles seen between positions: e.g. a prop forward and wing back in rugby, a wicket keeper and fast bowler in cricket, a linebacker and wide receiver in American football.

### Training errors

As discussed earlier, athletes may do too much, too soon, and too frequently. Training errors are one of the commonest causes of chronic overuse injuries, and practitioners must identify these errors for successful treatment planning. Failure to do so will lead to a recurrence of the injury or development of other overuse injuries. To avoid injury athletes who wish to exercise regularly must find the correct balance of exercise intensity, duration and frequency. This will normally involve:

- participating in more than one sport
- combination of strength, flexibility and endurance training
- incorporation of rest days in the weekly training schedule
- periods during the year of greater training/sport levels, i.e. seasons
- variation in training methods to help maintain interest.

When athletes first begin to train they often overestimate their baseline fitness level. This can result in injury, as the musculoskeletal system is not physiologically prepared for this volume of exercise. Common injuries at this stage are muscle strains and exercise-induced leg pain (shin splints). Increasing the volume of exercise too quickly can also occur when an athlete is returning from injury or training for a specific competition that they are not prepared for.

Bones, like muscle, also undergo a normal physiological strengthening process during the early period of an exercise programme. This remodelling process is characterised by initial bone porosity due to osteoclastic channelling, which is then followed by osteoblasts laying down new bone matrix. The result is that the bone is initially weakened by exercise and then eventually strengthened beyond its pre-exercise level.

# CAUSES OF PAIN IN THE FOOT

## ARTICULAR AND BONE CONDITIONS

### Osteoarthritis (OA)

Degenerative arthritis may affect any of the joints of the foot and ankle. The joints most commonly affected are the ankle, subtalar, calcaneocuboid, talonavicular, first tarsometatarsal and first metatarsophalangeal joint (MTPJ). The first MTPJ will be considered separately under the heading of hallux rigidus.

*Aetiology*

This may be primary with no known cause but, while such arthritis is common in the hip and knee, it is rare in the ankle. Far more commonly OA is secondary to some insult to the joint and may follow major injury, such as a fracture extending into the joint, a dislocation or repeated minor trauma. Fractures of the neck of the talus may also lead to OA of the ankle. Other causes can include:

- *Infection in the joint.* Septic arthritis, unless diagnosed and treated early, will lead to lysis of cartilage and secondary OA.

- *Inflammatory arthropathies* such as rheumatoid arthritis (RA) and the seronegative arthritides, e.g. psoriatic arthritis, Reiter's disease and ankylosing spondylitis.
- *Metabolic disorders* such as gout and pseudogout.
- *Systemic diseases* such as diabetes mellitus, which can lead to Charcot foot or ankle; the ankle is affected in about 10% of Charcot foot cases.
- *Proximal malalignment*, e.g. following a malunited fractured tibia, has frequently been stated to lead to arthritis by imposing abnormal stresses on distal joints. While some authors have allowed up to 10° in the sagittal or frontal plane (Nicoll 1964), others have felt that even a few degrees of angulation may lead to significant problems (Johnson 1987). Merchant disputed this in a long-term follow-up study when he could find no correlation between the degree of malunion and the occurrence of OA (Merchant & Dietz 1989).
- *Other miscellaneous conditions* such as haemophilia or avascular necrosis (Freiberg's disease affecting second metatarsal head).

*Presenting symptoms*

Generally these will be pain and stiffness in the area of the affected joint. Symptoms may start as

**Table 16.2**  The four basic domains of foot health as evaluated by the Foot Health Status Questionnaire (FHSQ)

| Domain | No. of items | Theoretical construct | Meaning of lowest score (0) | Meaning of highest score (100) |
|---|---|---|---|---|
| Foot pain | 4 | Evaluation of foot pain in terms of type of pain, severity and duration | Extreme and significant foot pain that is acute in nature | No pain or discomfort in any part of the foot |
| Foot function | 4 | Evaluation of feet in terms of impact on physical function | Severely limited in performing a broad range of physical activities because of feet: limited in walking, working and moving about | Can perform all desired physical activities: walking, working and climbing stairs |
| Footwear | 3 | Lifestyle issues related to footwear and feet | Extremely limited in access to suitable footwear | No problems with obtaining suitable footwear |
| General foot health | 2 | Self-perception of feet (individual's subjective assessment of body image related to feet) | Generally perceives feet to be in a poor state of health and identifies poor condition of feet | Perceives feet to be in an excellent state of health and condition |

aching after exercise and progress of pain after walking a distance. With time and progression of the arthritis the distance the patient can walk without pain gradually reduces. Pain may become constant and also present at night, disturbing sleep. How much pain the patient is experiencing is important to know but quantifying pain is difficult, because individual patients will have different tolerances to pain and different attitudes to the degree of their disability. While one can ask the patient to quantify their pain on a visual analogue scale of, say, 1–10, it is function which probably influences us most when it comes to determining treatment. While one must beware the stoic who pushes himself on regardless of the pain (and vice versa), how much a patient can do is often a good indicator of how severe the symptoms are. Stiffness may initially occur after the joint has been rested for a while, but with time the range of movement in the affected joint will decrease. Dorsiflexion is usually the first movement to be lost, and shoes with a slight heel raise may therefore be more comfortable. In severe OA the joint may completely lose movement and become virtually ankylosed. Patients may also complain of a limp, swelling or joint deformity.

### Signs

The joint may appear swollen or deformed or be held in an abnormal position. The joint may feel warm if the underlying cause is infection or an inflammatory arthropathy, but otherwise not. An effusion may be present in ankle OA but is not usually clinically detectable in OA of other foot joints. Osteophytes may be felt in superficial joints as hard bony swellings and represent new bone formation around the periphery of affected joints. Localised tenderness may also be found. The range of movement of the joint will be reduced, the degree depending on how advanced the arthritis is, and movement will be painful, more so at extremes. Often movement may feel 'dry', rather than smooth and easy. In advanced OA grating or crunching may be felt by the examiner as the joint is moved.

### Investigations

Plain X-rays, generally standing anteroposterior (AP for ankle, DP (dorsiplantar) for foot) and lateral, are essential (Ch. 11). The cardinal signs of OA are reduced joint space, sclerosis, cysts and osteophytes (see Fig. 11.27). Standing films are helpful as they may demonstrate deformity under load and the true loss of joint space due to cartilage erosion. Special views may be helpful to show the subtalar joint; Anthonsen's view shows the medial and posterior subtalar facets. If infection is suspected then any open wounds can be swabbed. Aspiration of the joint to obtain bacteriology may be helpful. Results from blood tests will be normal and are unhelpful unless the OA is secondary to a systemic disease, infection or metabolic cause such as gout (Ch. 13). Further to the discussion on pain it should be noted that the degree of X-ray change does not always correlate in a linear fashion with the patient's symptoms or disability. It is always important to treat the patient and not the X-ray.

### Differential diagnosis

In early OA, when X-rays are normal, a presumptive diagnosis may be made solely on information from the history, symptoms and signs. Other periarticular causes should be considered however. In established OA, with X-ray changes, the differential diagnosis will usually lie in determining the underlying cause.

## Footballer's ankle

### Aetiology

This condition was well described by McMurray in 1950 and occurs in soccer players as a result of repeated kicking of the ball with the foot held in equinus (McMurray 1950). In this position the anterior capsule largely takes the strain, as the extensor tendons are mechanically disadvantaged, and bony traction spurs develop.

### Presenting symptoms

These will be pain, often on kicking a stationary ball, but also on dorsiflexion of the ankle. The

## Signs

At rest physical examination may be normal, although there may be some tenderness over the distal tibia. This may become more marked if the patient exercises on a treadmill to produce symptoms.

## Investigations

Plain X-rays should be taken to exclude a stress fracture or other osseous causes of leg pain. Measuring compartment pressures with a catheter introduced under local anaesthetic is the most useful way to confirm the diagnosis.

Pressures are measured before and after exercise. There is some debate as to the correct abnormal compartment pressures. Generally, intracompartmental pressures at rest should be less than 15 mmHg and 5–10 min following exercise should have returned to 15 mmHg or less (Pedowitz et al 1990).

## Differential diagnosis

Shin splints or stress fractures of the tibia will be the main differential diagnosis for leg pains. For neurological symptoms in the foot an entrapment neuropathy should be excluded.

## NERVES

A number of nerves may be compressed at sites around the ankle and foot, resulting in entrapment neuropathies.

## Tarsal tunnel syndrome

### Aetiology

The posterior tibial nerve, a branch of the sciatic nerve, may become compressed as it passes under the flexor retinaculum behind the medial malleolus (Fig. 16.10). Interestingly, tarsal tunnel syndrome is a relatively new diagnosis, having only been properly first described in 1962 (Keck 1962, Lam 1962). The condition is analogous to carpal tunnel syndrome in the wrist but nowhere near as common. The com-

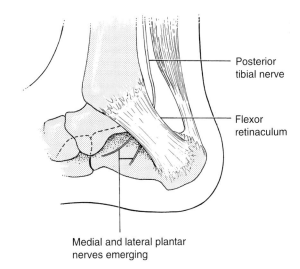

**Figure 16.10** Line drawing to show gross anatomy of the tarsal tunnel – lateral view.

pression may cause direct pressure, leading to motor and sensory symptoms, or may compress the vascular supply, the vasa nervorum, causing sensory symptoms only. Aetiology of tarsal tunnel syndrome is idiopathic, trauma or associated with bony alignment (Cimino 1990). Other cases may be related to problems such as rheumatoid arthritis or compression within the tunnel associated with a ganglion, lipoma or venous varicosities.

### Presenting symptoms

The patient is likely to complain of a diffuse, burning type of pain on the sole of the foot. With time symptoms may become more localised. Often pain is worse on activity and better at rest. A proportion of patients get night-time pain and some 30% have proximal radiation of pain to the midcalf region, known as the Valleix phenomenon (Mann 1993).

### Signs

Sensory or motor weakness is rare to find but should be carefully looked for. Most useful is a positive Tinel sign, obtained by starting proximally and percussing along the course of the nerve. At the site of entrapment percussion will cause radiation of pain along the course of the nerve.

## Investigations

Plain X-rays may demonstrate any post-traumatic bony spurs causing compression but do not in themselves make a diagnosis. Electrodiagnostic tests are necessary for this: nerve conduction studies looking at sensory conduction velocities and the amplitude and duration of motor-evoked potentials (Ch. 7). Tests should be performed bilaterally and a peripheral neuropathy should be excluded. If an extrinsic compression in the tunnel is suspected then an MRI may be helpful.

## Differential diagnosis

Because of the diffuse nature of the symptoms the differential diagnosis is quite wide, but two possibilities should be particularly looked for. A peripheral neuropathy, e.g. from diabetes, may cause burning pains in the foot, but is usually bilateral. Sciatica with nerve root irritation causing distal pain also needs to be excluded. Straight leg raising will be restricted and painful.

# Other entrapments

## Aetiology

Other entrapments which have been described include the deep peroneal nerve under the inferior extensor retinaculum and the superficial peroneal nerve as it exits the deep fascia about 11.5 cm above the lateral malleolus, the medial plantar nerve at the master knot of Henry and the first branch of the lateral plantar nerve between abductor hallucis and quadratus plantae muscles. Most of these entrapments occur in runners or athletes.

## Symptoms and signs

**Deep peroneal nerve.** Patients complain of pain over the dorsum of the foot and sometimes numbness and paraesthesia in the first web space. There may be altered sensation in the first web space and a positive Tinel sign.

**Superficial peroneal nerve.** Symptoms include pain over the dorsum of the foot and ankle and inferior lateral border of the calf. As a sensory nerve there are no motor signs but there may be a positive Tinel sign. A fascial defect or muscle herniation where the nerve exits the deep fascia should be looked for.

**Medial plantar nerve.** Patients complain of an aching pain over the medial aspect of the arch, often radiating into the medial three toes, becoming worse on running. Again, a positive Tinel sign may be found and also tenderness under the medial arch (Case history 16.4).

**First branch of lateral plantar nerve.** Patients complain of chronic pain, often increased on running but sometimes present on waking. On examination there will be tenderness over the nerve deep to abductor hallucis and pressure reproduces the patient's symptoms.

## Investigations

Nerve conduction studies may help with the diagnosis of deep peroneal nerve entrapment, but are less useful in diagnosing the others. More

---

**Case history 16.4**

**Patient:** 48-year-old keen runner; squash and badminton player.

**Presenting symptoms:** 18-month history of bilateral paraesthesia affecting the medial aspect of the soles of both feet, in the distribution of the medial plantar nerve, when running. Symptoms initially settled after exercise but over the next 6 months the patient developed shooting pains without any pattern of onset with increasing numbness in both feet.

**Signs:** A positive Tinel sign above both medial malleoli. Some loss of sharp and blunt sensory discrimination on the medial aspect of the sole was identified.

**Investigations:** Nerve conduction studies showed conduction blocks bilaterally at the level of the tarsal tunnel. Medial plantar responses were absent on the right and delayed on the left.

**Diagnosis:** Bilateral tarsal tunnel syndrome.

**Operative findings:** On both sides there was a high division of the posterior tibial nerve into medial and lateral plantar branches. A sharp edge to abductor hallucis was found to be compressing the medial plantar nerve bilaterally. In addition there was a large vascular pedicle crossing the medial plantar nerve and compressing it more proximally. Pain settled following surgery.

recently, abnormalities of nerve conduction and electromyography have demonstrated plantar nerve abnormalities (Schon et al 1993). Injection of local anaesthetic at the site of entrapment may act as a diagnostic test if it abolishes symptoms.

### Differential diagnosis

As for tarsal tunnel syndrome.

## Peripheral neuropathy

### Aetiology

Peripheral neuropathies may be due to a variety of causes. In the West the leading cause is diabetes and in the Third World it is leprosy. Other causes include spina bifida, pernicious anaemia, drugs and alcoholism. The different patterns of peripheral neuropathy may vary but in diabetics the most common is a symmetrical distal polyneuropathy, encompassing motor, sensory and autonomic components.

### Presenting symptoms

Patients may notice no symptoms at all if the neuropathy presents as a painless one. The first inkling of a problem may be when a patient presents with a complication such as ulceration or infection. In a diabetic who normally has a painless foot with no sensation the presence of pain is important and may indicate deep infection, such as an abscess or osteomyelitis. If the presentation is of a painful neuropathy the patient may complain of a burning sensation in the legs and feet, commonly worse at night.

### Signs

In a diabetic the foot may adopt a cavus appearance with clawed toes. In the absence of vascular disease the foot will feel warm and there may be distended veins. Sensation to light touch and pinprick will be reduced and joint position sense may be impaired. The toes may be clawed with wasting of the intrinsic foot muscles and the ankle jerk absent. Callosities may be present under the metatarsal heads and heel.

### Investigations

In evaluating a peripheral neuropathy it is important to look for an underlying cause. The urine should be tested for sugar and a random blood glucose test performed to look for the most common cause. A careful history and examination should uncover evidence of other causes. Nerve conduction studies may be helpful to rule out an entrapment neuropathy.

## Morton's metatarsalgia (neuroma)

### Aetiology

This condition is a type of entrapment neuropathy affecting a plantar digital nerve. It most commonly affects the common digital nerve to the 3/4 interspace, but may also occur in the 2/3 interspace. The diagnosis probably does not exist in the first or fourth webspaces, although there has been much debate about this. The incidence of a second neuroma in the same foot is 4% (Thompson & Deland 1993). Women are affected at least four times more often than men and the condition can affect adults of any age. The nerve develops a fusiform swelling, just proximal to its bifurcation, at the level of the intermetatarsal bursa (Fig. 16.11). Although frequently termed a neuroma, technically it is not as the histology shows a degenerative process rather than a proliferative one.

### Presenting symptoms

The patient complains of a burning pain on the sole of the foot, at the level of the metatarsal heads and commonly radiating into one or two toes. It may feel to the patient like walking on a sharp pebble. Occasionally, pain will radiate proximally. Pain is often worse on walking and may be particularly exacerbated by tight-fitting shoes, as these will compress the metatarsal heads together, thus 'trapping' the nerve. Resting or removing tight shoes may settle the pain. Less than half the patients complain of numbness in the toes.

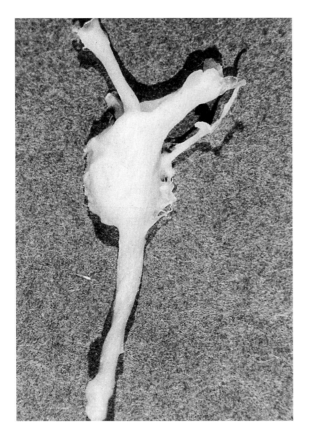

**Figure 16.11**  Resected Morton's neuroma showing terminal digital branches following operation.

### Signs

On palpation of the relevant interspace the patient's pain will be reproduced, sometimes with radiation into a toe. However, it may be difficult to elicit conclusive evidence on examination. If pressure is maintained in the interspace with one hand, while the other alternately squeezes the forefoot from side to side to compress the metatarsal heads together, then a painful click may be obtained. This is known as Mulder's click and is only helpful if it reproduces pain (Mulder 1951). It is important to ensure that any tenderness is not over the metatarsal heads, rather than intermetatarsal, although in rare cases nerves may become entrapped under a metatarsal head. Sensation in the toes is usually normal, but may vary.

### Investigations

Plain X-rays should be taken to rule out other pathology. Although ultrasound and MRI have been used to look for the swelling in the nerve they have not generally proved reliable enough to be used as diagnostic tools. Ultrasound has been reported as useful if the neuroma is 5 mm in diameter (Pollak et al 1992). Nerve conduction studies are not helpful. A diagnostic injection of local anaesthetic may be helpful if it abolishes the patient's pain.

### Differential diagnosis

Problems affecting the metatarsal head, such as synovitis, intermetatarsal bursa and Freiberg's disease, should be considered. It is important to be careful about whether the tenderness is under a metatarsal head or intermetatarsal. Pain from a neurological cause, such as tarsal tunnel syndrome, peripheral neuropathy or referred pain from the back should be excluded.

## SKIN AND SUBCUTANEOUS TISSUES

## Retrocalcaneal bursitis

### Aetiology

There are two bursae at the heel; one is deep to the tendo Achilles and the other lies superficial to its insertion. The deep bursa is infrequently affected but, as it has a synovial lining, symptoms may be early indicators of an inflammatory arthropathy such as rheumatoid arthritis. Men are affected more often than women. Symptoms in the subcutaneous bursa affect adolescent females most frequently.

### Presenting symptoms

For the subcutaneous bursa the symptoms are well described by some of the eponyms for the condition, sucha as 'pump or heel bumps'. The patient complains of a tender prominence at the heel when wearing shoes (Fig. 16.12).

also used to indicate the degree of risk, the number of possible factors increases further, making the designing of an easy-to-use system all the harder.

The second task is to obtain clear definitions of these factors. The lack of universal consensus on definitions makes comparison difficult. For example, a very simple classification system of ulcers which nonetheless is an aid to prognosis and degree of risk, is to determine whether the ulcer is superficial or deep. However, unless there are clear definitions as to exactly what is understood by these two terms, we cannot be sure that an ulcer graded as superficial by one practitioner, which subsequently deteriorates, would not have been classified as deep by another.

Thirdly, an accurate but simple means is needed to measure the factors concerned, and such means are not available for all factors. For example, it is generally held that if an ulcer can be probed to bone, it is assumed that osteomyelitis is present, regardless of whether it can be detected on X-ray, but this rule has not been validated by research.

Similar problems apply to the presence of ischaemia and neuropathy (Chs 6 and 7).

So far, no single system has been designed which is appropriate to all situations: each has its limitations and many practitioners will use a combination of classification and description to record both details of loss of tissue viability and to estimate the degree of risk.

## Aetiological classification

One example of a well-validated classification system for lower limb ulcers is the aetiological system (Table 17.3). This is appropriate for use by practitioners in a clinical setting as it is a useful guide for a treatment plan, since removal or amelioration of the cause will be a fundamental step in the treatment. There is also some correlation between cause and prognosis, e.g. an uncomplicated neuropathic ulcer has a significantly better prognosis than a similar-sized ischaemic ulcer. Although used more often for the classification of ulcers, this system can be easily adapted to classify loss of tissue viability. The precise categories

**Table 17.3** An example of an aetiological system of classification of lower limb ulcers

| Category of lesion | Examples of conditions |
| --- | --- |
| Dermatological | Atopic eczema |
| Endocrine | Diabetes mellitus |
| Haematological | Sickle-cell anaemia, cryoglobulinaemia |
| Iatrogenic | Stevens–Johnson syndrome |
| Immunological | Rheumatoid arthritis |
| Infectious | Tuberculosis |
| Neoplastic | Squamous cell carcinoma, malignant melanoma, Kaposi's sarcoma, basal cell carcinoma |
| Neurological | Hansen's disease (leprosy), diabetes mellitus, syringomyelia |
| Traumatic | Burns, friction blisters, cuts, pressure sores |
| Vascular | Peripheral vascular disease, venous hypertension |

can be altered according to the wishes of the practitioner. For example, vascular could be divided into arterial, venous and lymphatic categories and iatrogenic could be included as a type of traumatic cause of ulceration.

It must be borne in mind that infection can complicate many lower limb ulcers, but is rarely a cause of ulceration. Nonetheless, this system has some limitations. It tells us nothing about the degree of loss of tissue viability. For this we could add a descriptive section, based on measurement of depth of the deepest part of the wound. This has been shown to have a strong correlation with prognosis and so would be helpful in determining the degree of risk of slow healing, ulceration and amputation. It is also possible that a particular lesion can be assigned to more than one category, which detracts from the precision of the system. For example, a basal cell carcinoma is a skin cancer and could be classified as both a neoplastic and a dermatological lesion and the ulcer seen in the diabetic foot could be classified as both endocrine and neurological.

**Meggit–Wagner wound classification system** (Table 17.4). This is another well-validated system which chiefly yields information as to the severity of the wound and therefore relates to prognosis and degree of risk. It has the further

**Table 17.4** Meggitt–Wagner wound classification

| Grade | Appearance | Implication |
|---|---|---|
| 1 | Loss of tissue involves dermis only | No significant ischaemic component |
| 2 | Loss exposes tendon or bone | |
| 3 | Loss exposes tendon or bone, with osteomyelitis or abscess | |
| 4 | Gangrene of digits or forefoot | Primarily an ischaemic problem |
| 5 | Extensive gangrene of the foot | |

advantage of dividing tissue loss into that with no significant ischaemic component and that where peripheral vascular disease is a major factor and so is of help in determining the most important steps in the subsequent treatment, since wounds which are primarily ischaemic will not heal unless steps are taken to improve the blood supply.

However, it has limitations, since it was designed to assess wounds and has no place for preulcerative conditions such as callus. This system has been adapted by some practitioners for the classification of loss of tissue viability by the addition of a grade 0 category for such conditions where no break in the epidermis has occurred. In addition, it would usually be expected that a patient with a grade 4 ulcer would have significant large-vessel disease of the lower limb and one would expect to find non-palpable pedal pulses. However, in patients with diabetes, it is quite possible for them to have digital gangrene and palpable pedal pulses, suggesting a grade 4 ulcer but with no significant major vessel pathology, the gangrene being a result of septic vasculitis or embolism. Small-vessel disease (i.e. thickening of the basement membrane) is no longer considered to be a prime cause of digital gangrene in patients with diabetes. Another limitation to this classification system is that there would be no place for the Charcot foot, even though this condition carries a high degree of risk of ulceration. A more detailed but similar classification system, which includes a grade 0 for intact skin and a separate grade for spreading infection, is the Sims classification (Sims et al 1988).

Almost all other systems are mainly descriptive and designed more to assess the degree of risk of ulceration/amputation than of classifying the ulcer per se. If they are to meet the criteria for simplicity and ease of use, they inevitably focus only on aetiological and local factors, e.g. *ischaemia and infection present*, which gives a limited view of factors contributing to risk.

**San Antonio/Texas System (Armstrong, Harkless and Lavery).** This group of practitioners designed two systems: one system is designed to classify the total range of loss of tissue viability, but has yet to be validated; the second system is concerned only with actual ulcers. The advantage of the first system is its comprehensiveness; both systems are an aid to prognosis and management.

The second system has been validated and grades ulcers according to depth, presence or absence of sepsis and presence or absence of ischaemia. No reference is made to the presence or absence of neuropathy however, which is considered by some practitioners as the single most important contributory factor to diabetic ulceration.

Using this system to assess the lesions of people with diabetes, Lavery et al (1996) were able to show that patients with infection and ischaemia were 90 times more likely to have an amputation than patients with lower-grade lesions, thus showing the importance of local wound conditions on outcome.

**S(AD) SAD system** (Table 17.5). This is a comprehensive system based on the San Antonio system but with modifications and extensions (Macfarlane & Jeffcoate 1999). It is also aimed at patients with diabetes but is designed for research and audit rather than as a guide to management. However, it could be adapted for management purposes (Serra 2000). The key elements of this system are size of a wound, as measured by both depth and surface area, infection, ischaemia and neuropathy. Each of these elements is assigned a grade from 0 to 3 according to severity, with grade 0 representing a normal foot and grade 3 representing the worst situation. The advantages of this

**Table 17.5**  The S(AD) SAD classification

| Grade | Area | Depth | Sepsis | Arteriopathy | Denervation |
|---|---|---|---|---|---|
| 0 | Skin intact | Skin intact | No infection | Pedal pulses palpable | Pinprick/VPT sensation normal |
| 1 | <10 mm$^2$ | Skin and subcutaneous tissues | Superficial: slough or exudates | Diminution of both pulses or absence of one | Reduced or absent pinprick sensation. VPT raised |
| 2 | 10–30 mm$^2$ | Tendon, joint capsule, periosteum | Cellulitis | Absence of both pedal pulses | Neuropathy dominant: palpable pedal pulses |
| 3 | >30 mm$^2$ | Bone and/or joint spaces | Osteomyelitis | Gangrene | Charcot foot |

system are that it covers the whole range of loss of tissue viability and includes the Charcot foot. However, the authors suggest testing *either* rather than *both* small and large nerve fibres for neuropathy which could lead to a false-negative result since denervation of each type of nerve fibre does not necessarily progress at the same rate. The measurement of the vibratory perception threshold requires the availability of a neurothesiometer for the latter, which may not be readily available in a routine clinic, but the authors do suggest the cheaper alternative method of using a 10 g monofilament. The authors acknowledge that measurement of neuropathy is an imperfect science. The system awaits full evaluation but there is a report of its successful use in a large multidisciplinary clinic in Portugal.

**Edmonds and Foster system.** This system is designed specifically to aid management of diabetic foot lesions by assigning the foot to a stage of graded severity, according to the criteria shown in Table 17.6, and dividing the lesions into one of two aetiological categories (neuropathic or neuroischaemic), as management differs for

**Table 17.6**  Staging the diabetic foot

| Stage | Clinical status |
|---|---|
| 1 | Normal. No presence of callus, ischaemia, neuropathy, deformity, swelling |
| 2 | High risk. One or more of the above is present |
| 3 | Skin breakdown or presence of blister, splits or grazes for more than 1 week |
| 4 | Ulcer and cellulitis |
| 5 | Necrosis |
| 6 | Advanced necrosis, foot cannot be saved |

these two categories. Edmonds & Forster (2000) acknowledge that their system of staging does not accommodate the Charcot foot and that the system would need extending for research and audit purposes.

## APPROACHES TO DETERMINING DEGREE OF RISK

### Holistic overview

To fully determine the degree of risk for any patient, one would need to take into account *all* factors which can influence healing, including not only the local condition of the lesion but also the patient and his environment. Although few of these latter factors are included in any proposed classification system, because such inclusion would make the system very cumbersome, much of the data will be recorded as part of a primary patient assessment (Ch. 5) and will be taken into account by the practitioner when assessing the degree of risk. Most work has been carried out on people with diabetes, as these people form the group with highest risk of worst-scenario lower limb complications of ulceration and non-traumatic amputation: 40–70% of all non-traumatic lower limb amputations are related to diabetes mellitus and 85% of all such amputations are preceded by a foot ulcer (International Working Group on the Diabetic Foot 1999).

### *Psychological factors*

Recent research has started to focus on patients' own perceptions of their health and their degree of risk. There is a strong association between non-compliance with therapy and amputation in a number of studies on patients with diabetes. The patient with diabetic neuropathy who has been told emphatically of the importance of checking his footwear and of the consequences of failure to heed this advice, but who returns later with an ulcer due to a foreign object in the shoe, possibly believes himself to be invulnerable: *it won't happen to me*. Education is seen as a vital part of the management of such patients, but simple transfer of knowledge is not enough. The patient's perception of his health status and the desire to alter behaviour are important influencing factors.

Complex interactions of psychological factors in people with at-risk feet can result in denial or detachment syndromes. In these cases patients perceive their foot health of low importance or relevance, often psychologically detaching themselves from their foot problems. These situations can be a particular challenge for practitioners to manage and call for a multiprofessional approach to assessment and management.

Other behavioural factors can be detrimental to health in general, such as tobacco smoking and excessive alcohol drinking, as well as having particular negative effects on healing outcomes.

### Socioeconomic factors

Low economic status has been shown to be associated with a higher risk of amputation. A person on a low income is less likely to be able to afford good footwear, adequate heating in the home, a balanced diet, etc. The socioeconomic status of an individual is more important than whether the person belongs to an ethnic minority group. Support in the form of family and friends and religious or social groups is important in reducing the risk, especially so in patients who suffer visual or other impairments, and this could be one reason why ethnic minorities are not at a disadvantage in terms of risk of lower limb ulceration and amputation. Lack of education in general is also an influencing factor: e.g. this may lead to inability to understand footcare advice or to realise the importance of adequate diet.

### Environmental factors

Reduced access to health care is also associated with increased risk. No matter how well motivated a patient may be, if there are inadequate footcare facilities, or those facilities are out of reach due to lack of transport, then there is always the possibility that a lesion will develop or worsen before adequate help is received. Other environmental factors such as inadequate heating in the home or poor hygiene are closely related to socioeconomic factors and lack of education, as discussed in the previous section.

### Occupational factors

Apart from the earnings-related factor, certain occupations independently place the person at a higher risk of lower limb complications. For example, people who have sedentary jobs are at higher risk of obesity, heart disease and venous stasis problems than people in more active jobs. People such as top executives who spend long hours in flight are also at high risk of deep vein thrombosis. Occupations involving exposure to the elements will increase that person's chance of developing cold-related conditions such as chilblains, which can lead to ulceration.

### Previous medical history

Past medical history is important, since previous ulceration or amputation will place the person in a high-risk category for further ulceration and amputation. This is because the factors that contributed to the development of the first ulcer are likely to still be present and, once amputation has been performed, the extra stress on the already compromised contralateral limb will place that limb at high risk.

### Age

The individual's healing ability will vary from person to person across any age band but in general healing slows with age. A more significant factor is the presence of coexistent disease, the likelihood of which increases with age.

## Coexistent disease

All too often a practitioner will be confronted with a non-healing ulcer: this, despite the fact that extreme care, the most appropriate dressings, antibiosis and careful observation and monitoring have all been carried out. In many such cases there is an underlying systemic condition which is delaying healing. There are many conditions which can delay healing and will therefore place the person in a higher risk category, some examples of which are shown in Table 17.7. In addition, the treatment itself for coexisting conditions may also impair healing.

A thorough primary patient assessment, as described in Chapters 5–10, should detect relevant underlying conditions/treatment.

## Local indicators

Having assessed the patient holistically for risk factors, it is necessary to turn our attention to the area of tissue viability loss itself and make an accurate recording of lesion details. This will often be carried out as part of the routine assessment of skin and the appendages in the clinic (Ch. 9). Some of the systems used have been discussed earlier in this chapter. Methods of obtaining descriptive details will now be discussed.

## Surface area of wound

The surface area of the wound is an important piece of data, since it enables the practitioner to chart the progress of a lesion and thus determine the success or otherwise of treatment.

Evidence of surface area as a prognosis for healing is contradictory, with a meta-analysis of wound healing studies by Margolis et al (2000) on diabetic neuropathic foot ulcers showing no correlation, whereas a recent paper by Oyibo et al (2001) looked at 194 patients with diabetic foot ulcers and found ulcer area at presentation was greater in the amputation group compared with healed ulcers, so the authors conclude that ulcer area does predict outcome and should be included in a wound classification system. The same authors found that the patient's age, sex, duration/type of diabetes, and ulcer site had no effect on outcome.

Methods of measuring surface area vary from the very simple to the very complicated.

The simplest method is to use a sterile, disposable millimetre ruler and record the longest axis of the wound as the length, $L$, and the width, $W$, as the longest dimension perpendicular to $L$. One of two formulae can then be used to calculate the surface area:

$$A = L \times W \times 0.785$$
or
$$A = L \times W \times 0.763$$

**Table 17.7**  Examples of conditions or treatments which may delay healing

| Category | Examples |
| --- | --- |
| Cardiovascular | Peripheral vascular disease, venous insufficiency, lymphatic obstruction |
| Endocrine/metabolic | Diabetes mellitus, malnutrition, deficiency syndromes, obesity |
| Immunological | DiGeorge syndrome, hypogammaglobulinaemia, human immunodeficiency virus, rheumatoid arthritis, hypersensitivity |
| Immunosuppressive agents | Long-term steroids, immunosuppressive drugs, radiation, cytotoxic drugs |
| Infectious | Cytomegalovirus, infectious mononucleosis, severe bacterial, mycobacterial or fungal disease |
| Haematological | Leukaemia, anaemias, haemophilia, sickle-cell anaemia |
| Musculoskeletal | Deformities, hypermobility |
| Neoplasia | Carcinomas, lymphomas, sarcomas |
| Respiratory | Chronic obstructive airways disease |
| Renal | Chronic nephropathy |
| Traumatic | Burns, foreign bodies, repeated minor trauma, tight clothing (tourniquet effect) |
| Exogenous factors | Inappropriate dressings, antiseptics, environmental conditions, caustics and irritants |

For derivations of these calculations, see Schubert (1997).

A second method requiring only simple apparatus is to place a sterile, flexible, transparent grid over the wound: the grid has a removable backing and is marked into 1-cm squares. The margins of the lesion can then be traced on to the grid and the surface area calculated by counting the squares. Disposal of the removable backing prevents cross-infection, and the tracing can be stored in the patient's notes for future reference. There are various strategies for calculation of surface area, such as including all whole squares and all partial squares on the right, discarding all partial squares on the left, etc., or using a formula such as:

$$A_C = N_C$$
$$A_{C+P} = (N_C + (0.4 \times N_P))$$

where $A_C$ is the surface area of whole squares, $A_{C+P}$ is the surface area of whole and partial squares, $N_C$ is the number of complete squares and $N_P$ is the number of partial squares within the traced area.

If the grid is divided into smaller squares, such as 0.5 cm × 0.5 cm then each formula has to be multiplied by 0.25 to obtain the area in cm$^2$ (Richard et al 2000).

Both of these methods have the advantage of being quick, simple to use and inexpensive. The disadvantages are that it is more difficult to obtain an accurate tracing if the lesion is on a curved surface such as the heel and that these methods are very subjective.

A more objective measurement is made by using a camera to take a photograph of the lesion. The camera must always be placed at a set distance from the lesion and a scaled ruler should be positioned at the top or bottom of the lesion, in the same vertical plane. The area of the lesion can then be calculated from the developed photograph. The advantages are that the measurement will be more objective and there is no risk of cross-infection, but disadvantages are that errors will again be present if the wound is on a curved surface, the equipment is much more expensive than use of a transparent grid and the result is not instantly available unless a Polaroid camera is used.

A further development is to use a digital camera and associated software, which will enable the image to be displayed on a computer screen. The operator can click on to various points around the margin of the lesion and the software will instantly calculate the surface area. The advantages are increased accuracy and instantaneous results. The disadvantages are the initial expense of the equipment and the need to develop a skill in operating the equipment.

A group of workers from France have developed a planimetry software program, which uses the tracing of the wound on a transparent grid together with the computer mouse acting as a digitiser, to transfer the tracing to the computer, whereupon the software automatically calculates the surface area. This method was compared with calculating the surface area by length and width, by square counting and by using image-processing software and was found to be highly reproducible and accurate. The advantage of this method is that it does not require the expense of a digital camera, but on the downside it is more time-consuming (Rajbhandari et al 1999).

### Depth of wound

The depth of the wound is an important piece of data, since as mentioned earlier, depth shows strong correlation with prognosis and degree of risk. The usual method is to use a blunt, sterile probe and measure the depth at the deepest part of the wound. The advantages are ease of use and low cost. The disadvantages are risk of cross-infection and deciding exactly where the deepest part of the lesion lies. It is also difficult to measure the depth of very narrow lesions such as fissures or splits in the epidermis. Lesions of unbroken skin will of course have zero depth.

### Volume of wound

Although some research is being undertaken using stereoscopic equipment, no very satisfactory method of measuring the volume of a wound has been developed. Other methods tried have included injecting normal saline and mea-

## REFERENCES

Armstrong D G, Lavery L A, Harkless L B 1998 Validation of a diabetic wound classfication system. Diabetes Care 21: 855–859

Carlson G L 1999 The influence of nutrition and sepsis upon wound healing. Journal of Wound Care 8: 471–474

Cotran R S, Kumar V, Robins S L 1994 Pathologic basis of disease. W B Saunders, Philadelphia, p 484

Edmonds M E, Foster A V M 2000 Managing the diabetic foot. Blackwell Science, Oxford, pp 3, 17–22

International Working Group on the Diabetic Foot 1999 International Consensus on the Diabetic Foot, pp 12, 66–67

Lavery L A, Armstrong D G, Harkless L B 1996 Classification of diabetic foot wounds. Journal of Foot and Ankle Surgery 35: 528–531

Macfarlane R M, Jeffcoate W J 1999 Classification of diabetic foot ulcers: the S(AD) SAD system. The Diabetic Foot 2: 123–131

Margolis D J, Kantor J, Berlin J A 2000 In: Boulton A J M, Connor H, Cavanagh P (eds) The foot in diabetes. John Wiley and Sons, Chichester, p 63

Mason J, O'Keefe C, McIntosh A, Hutchinson A, Booth A, Young R J 1999 A systematic review of foot ulcers in patients with type 2 diabetes mellitus. 1: prevention. Diabetic Medicine 16: 801–812

Oyibo S O, Jude E B, Tarawneh I et al 2001 The effects of ulcer size and site, patient's age, sex and type and duration of diabetes on the outcome of diabetic foot ulcers. Diabetic Medicine 18: 133–138

Rajbhandari S, Harris N D, Sutton M et al 1999 Digital imaging: an accurate and easy method of measuring foot ulcers. Diabetic Medicine 16: 339–342

Richard J L, Daures J P, Parer-Richard C, Vannereau D, Boulot I 2000 Wounds 12: 148–154

Schubert V 1997 Measuring the area of chronic ulcers for consistent documentation in clinical practice. Wounds 9: 153–159

Serra L 2000 Clinic currently testing the S(AD) SAD classification system – letters. The Diabetic Foot 3: 10

Sims D S, Cavanagh, Ulbrecht J S 1988 Risk factors in the diabetic foot. Recognition and management. Physical Therapy 68: 1887–1902

Young M 2000 Classification of ulcers and its relevance to management. In: Boulton A J M, Connor H, Cavanagh P (eds) The foot in diabetes. John Wiley and Sons, Chichester, pp 61–62

## FURTHER READING

Banks V 1998 Wound assessment methods. Journal of Wound Care 7: 211–212

Letters 2000 The Diabetic Foot 3: 42

# 18

# Assessment of the elderly

*W. Turner*

## INTRODUCTION

The majority of people seeking advice for foot problems are over the age of 65 years. Surveys of podiatry caseloads identify people over this age as the largest consumers of foot health services. As the population ages, so the demands on providers of foot health services are likely to increase. It is, therefore, essential for elderly people to receive a structured and systematic assessment of their foot/lower limb problem if effective care is to be provided.

Whereas the general principles of assessment of the lower limb apply to the elderly, there are some particular considerations which practitioners need to consider when assessing the elderly. Growing old is sometimes perceived as a disease process. However, unlike a disease, growing old is an inevitable, time-dependent process which will occur to all individuals, providing that life is not prematurely ended. Ageing is therefore an unstoppable process for which there is no escape or cure. The role of the practitioner is, therefore, to minimise the effects of age-related degeneration of body systems, and to enable the elderly to compensate for such changes.

The aim of any intervention is to enable the elderly person to continue to meet the challenges presented to them by their particular environments and circumstances. For example, a painful bunion joint may prevent an elderly person walking to the shops. Appropriate foot care provision may relieve the patient's pain and improve physical function, thereby enabling the patient to walk to the shops without pain and discomfort. Even relatively simple foot problems, such as neglected long toe nails, can limit an individual's ability to cope with the demands of daily living. Nail problems may prevent a person from wearing outdoor shoes, and therefore restrict the person's living environment to their home. Such confinement can result in social isolation, causing further health deterioration and severe reductions to the quality of life.

## ASSESSMENT OF THE ELDERLY POPULATION

The size of the elderly population has increased over the last century. For example, in the United Kingdom, the number of people of pensionable age has risen from 2 million in 1901 to 10 million in 2001 – Office for Census and Population Statistics (OPCS) data. In the UK, the over 65s now make up around 20% of the general population. Reasons for improved longevity include improved water and sewage treatment, better nutrition, improvements in housing and better social and economic circumstances. The impact of improvements in medical care on average life span is less quantifiable.

Community podiatry services predominantly provide foot health services to people over the age of 65 years. In 1997 a total of 975 000 new referrals were made to NHS podiatry services in the United Kingdom. Of these, 63% (614 250) were for people aged 65 years or over (Hansard 1998). In the same year, a total of 9 million face-to-face contacts were carried out by community podiatry services, costing a total of £99.6 million (US$149 million).

The prevalence of foot morbidity amongst elderly populations is difficult to determine. There have been relatively few studies which have quantified foot morbidity amongst the elderly. In those surveys of foot morbidity which have been published, the most commonly reported foot problems amongst the elderly were difficulties with nail cutting, corns and hard skin, respectively (Crawford et al 1995). In the same survey, around half of people over the age of 75 years complained of two or more foot problems.

A recent meta-analysis of the literature shows forecast prevalence data for foot pathologies for populations over the age of 65 years (Table 18.1). However, this does not include studies of high-risk groups (e.g. people with diabetes) and probably underestimates the true prevalence of foot conditions in general populations. The large standard deviations and confidence intervals for many of the pathologies reviewed demonstrate the relatively high variation of reported prevalence of foot disease in the literature. Nevertheless, these data can be used to provide a rough estimate of foot morbidity for a given population.

There is certainly evidence that the likelihood of experiencing foot problems, and the likely need for community foot health services, increases with advancing age. This is particularly true for elderly women, who are the largest consumers of UK NHS podiatry services (Harvey et al 1997).

**Table 18.1** Forecast prevalence of foot pathologies amongst the elderly population (from Turner et al 2001)

| Condition | Mean prevalence | 95% confidence interval | Standard deviation |
|---|---|---|---|
| Hyperkeratosis | 54.88 | 47.78, 61.98 | 11.46 |
| Hypertrophic nails | 39.8 | 19.76, 59.84 | 14.42 |
| Toe deformity | 30.68 | 9.91, 51.45 | 23.64 |
| Onychomycosis | 40 | 16.77, 63.23 | 23.7 |
| Hallux deformity | 23.14 | 14.77, 31.51 | 9.56 |
| Diminished sensation | 19.83 | 14.69, 24.97 | 4.54 |
| Vascular insufficiency | 16.98 | 10.4, 23.56 | 7.52 |
| Poor foot hygiene | 20.9 | 4.99, 36.81 | 11.45 |
| Foot ulceration | 4.15 | 0, 8.36 | 3.04 |

people, respiratory problems seen in combination with other coexisting disorders present the greatest threat. For example, elderly people with emphysema coupled with peripheral vascular disease may suffer ulceration of the foot. In this example, the reduction in oxygenation of the blood may complicate an already compromised tissue viability.

## Functional assessment of the elderly

Functional assessment of the elderly patient is an important part of the assessment process. A good functional assessment will provide the practitioner with a clear impression of a patient's capabilities and limitations and identify the effect of lower limb disorders on lifestyle. It will also assist with risk assessment of the elderly person.

Table 18.7 details aspects of functional assessment which may be included as part of the general assessment of the elderly patient.

Assessment of function before and after clinical intervention can be a useful means for the determination of clinical effectiveness. Some of the key therapeutic objectives for managing lower limb pathology in the elderly are concerned with the following:

1. maintaining or improving the patient's independence
2. improving the patient's mobility
3. improving the patient's quality of life
4. enabling the patient to undertake activities of daily living (ADLs).

These objectives are as important as disease/symptom specific objectives (e.g. reducing pain). Therapeutic interventions which have an effect on the above will often make a significant difference to the patient. This is true even where cure of the presenting problem is not possible. Most patients are more concerned about reductions in functional ability and becoming dependent on others (i.e. becoming a 'burden') than anything else.

An inter-professional approach to therapy can be particularly useful to the assessment of function. Physiotherapists and occupational therapists, for example, make use of a variety of func-

**Table 18.7**  Examples of functional assessments of the elderly patient

| | |
|---|---|
| Independence | What are the patient's capabilities? Can the patient carry out activities of daily living without assistance? Is the patient adequately compensating for the effects of disease? Can the patient adjust to changes in her environment? What does the patient need the help of other people to do? What does the patient's social network consist of? |
| Mobility | Is the patient able to move around her environment without assistance? Does the patient drive? Can the patient climb stairs safely? Can the patient manage to do her own shopping, visit hairdresser, chemist, doctor, etc.? Does the patient require special aids to assist her mobility (e.g. stick, frame, wheelchair)? Is the patient stable when standing or walking? Is the patient likely to fall? |
| Activities of daily living | What activities does the patient feel she needs to do on a daily basis? Can the patient cope with feeding and grooming herself? Can the patient dress/undress independently? Can the patient manage to cut her own toe nails and/or apply creams to the feet? Can the patient maintain a clean and hygienic home? |
| Quality of life | Is the patient satisfied with her life? Is the patient happy or sad? Is the patient lonely or isolated? Does the patient keep herself occupied? Are there things which the patient enjoys doing? Does the patient feel guilty about anything? Is the patient worried, frightened or concerned? Is the patient experiencing painful symptoms? Does the patient feel that physical disease or pain is affecting her lifestyle? |
| Cognitive state | Is the patient confused? Is the patient forgetful? Can the patient describe her symptoms? Is the patient capable of giving informed consent? |

tional assessment strategies which can provide the practitioner with useful information as part of an overall assessment of the patient.

Functional assessment often focuses on the following:

- mobility and independence
- quality of life
- ability to perform ADLs.

In addition, there are other functional assessments which may be particularly relevant to the lower limb:

- gait analysis
- ability to self-care for feet.

The most popular means of assessing mobility and independence is the Barthel index. This was first developed by Mahoney & Barthel (1965) for the assessment of long-stay hospital patients with neuromuscular or musculoskeletal problems. It has since been used for the assessment of community- (home-) based patients with a variety of pathologies. The index is designed for the assessment of function both before and after treatment. It is therefore useful for the determination of the efficacy of clinical intervention. Table 18.8 shows the key elements of the Barthel index.

The Barthel index does not include some important activities of daily living such as shopping, cooking, social activities and gardening, which probably reflects the fact that the index was originally designed to assess institutionalised populations.

Deterioration in independence and mobility usually progresses through:

1. Social activities of daily living – i.e. how the person relates to the 'outside world' – e.g. shopping, visiting friends and relatives, vacations, going to the pub, etc.

2. Domestic activities of daily living – i.e. how the person manages household tasks – e.g. cooking, cleaning, gardening, etc.
3. Personal activities of daily living – i.e. how the person manages to care for herself – e.g. washing, bathing, cutting toe nails, continence, etc.

Therefore, an elderly person will usually experience difficulty with visiting the shops before having problems with cooking or bathing. Similarly, incontinence usually occurs later on after the person has developed other functional limitations. This can make continence a particularly difficult situation to manage for both the patient and carers. Many other factors often contribute to the onset of incontinence, including loss of mobility, urinary tract infection, autonomic neuropathy, prostatism, stress incontinence, unstable bladder, retention with overflow and central nervous system (CNS) pathology.

There are a variety of means to test an individual's mobility. A simple mobility assessment is known as the 'timed up and go' test. In this test, the elderly person is asked to stand from a chair, walk 10 feet, turn and return to the chair. The person is timed during this activity. Most adults can complete this activity in less than 10 seconds. Frail elderly people may take from 11 to 20 seconds for this task. People taking longer than 20 seconds are generally amongst the most immobile elderly. For this latter group a more detailed mobility assessment is indicated. There is a strong association between the results of this test and a person's functional independence in activities of daily living.

**Table 18.8** Key aspects of Barthel index

Feeding
Mobility (from bed to chair)
Personal toilet (washing, etc.)
Getting on/off toilet
Bathing
Walking on a level surface
Going up/down stairs
Dressing
Continence (bladder/bowel)

## Assessment of gait in the elderly

Assessment of gait in the elderly patient can often be a useful indicator of mobility. It can also enable the practitioner to determine whether walking aids (e.g. sticks, frame) are indicated. A reduction in walking speed is one of the early features of gait disturbance in the elderly. Healthy adult cadence is about 1 m/s. A frail elderly person may walk at less than half this speed.

Elderly stride length is often shorter than that of a younger adult. Gait is often apropulsive, with limited toe-off evident. This appears as a 'shuffling' gait. The base of gait is often wide, in an attempt to improve balance and stability. The elderly person may grasp fixed objects to improve stability. In this way, elderly people often use objects around their room to move around safely. This is especially common for elderly people with sight problems.

Frail elderly people placed in an unfamiliar environment will often show a much slower and more 'unsure' gait than they would normally have at home. Lack of familiar objects for stability or an unfamiliar walking surface can cause perceptual problems and lack of confidence. Therefore, asking an elderly person to walk down a long corridor in a hard-floored clinic can give an unrepresentative picture of the person's gait. Gait is best observed in an environment which is familiar to the patient (e.g. home).

Peripheral sensory neuropathy may produce a 'high stepping' gait with a characteristically heavy heel strike. Parkinson's disease produces a 'festinating' gait where the person appears to chase their centre of gravity forwards, shuffling and stooping. Musculoskeletal problems, joint pain or foot pain can result in an antalgic (pain-avoiding) gait. This often manifests as limping or avoiding certain movements or positions of the limb during gait.

## Determinants of the quality of life

Quality of life is affected by a complex interaction of multiple factors, some of which can have a large impact on quality of life (Table 18.9).

There are many measurement tools for the assessment of quality of life. The most popular tool used in UK health care for the assessment of quality of life in studies of adults with disease states is the short form-36 questionnaire (SF-36). The SF-36 questionnaire consists of 36 questions divided into the following categories: physical health, physiological health, mental health and social well-being. Its popularity has resulted in a large number of studies which are able to attest

**Table 18.9**   Major factors affecting quality of life

Loss of mobility
Dependence on others
Acute or chronic pain
General health status
Life-threatening/ terminal disease
Poverty
Social isolation
Loneliness
Mental state – e.g. depression
Bereavement
Difficulty sleeping
Boredom
Inability to perform activities of daily living
Loss of ability to make decisions
Lack of control

the validity and reliability of the questionnaire for a wide variety of clinical situations.

The SF-36 assessment tool is available free of charge from the UK Clearing House for Information on the Assessment of Health Outcomes, Nuffield Institute for Health Service Studies (see References for web site address).

More informal assessment of the quality of life of the elderly can be achieved through normal clinical conversation. The practitioner, as part of a normal discussion with the patient, can gain a fair idea of the patient's quality of life. Podiatry is a profession which is well suited to this task, since patients are often seated for treatment for 20 min or so, and treatment does not usually prevent the patient from talking. Patient and podiatrist are usually sitting face to face, and one-to-one communication is established. Where a podiatrist is concerned that the patient has a poor quality of life, or feels that the patient is unusually sad or depressed, a more formal assessment of quality of life can be undertaken. This may involve a referral to other members of the health and social care team: e.g. health visitor, social worker or general practitioner (GP).

## Assessment of cognitive status

Assessment of cognitive function in the elderly can be important for all health care workers.

This is particularly important where a practitioner seeks informed consent from a patient for a clinical procedure. Those changes most frequently associated with the ageing process are forgetfulness and confusion. Forgetfulness is a behaviour which affects all people, young or old. The fact that elderly people appear to forget things more often may be related to several factors. First, people who are old today received a different education to people who are young today. Some elderly people will have received a very basic education, had poor schooling and, as a result, may appear less intelligent and more forgetful. Coupled with this is the fact that most elderly people had limited exposure to the media when they were young compared with young people today who are exposed to a mass media. This cohort effect is probably an important factor in explaining why elderly people have difficulty remembering certain facts, recalling events and handling complex ideas. It is important to remember that forgetfulness is not necessarily indicative of the onset of brain disease or dementia.

Dementia is another cause of forgetfulness. It is a relatively common finding in elderly people. Dementia can arise as a result of reductions in supply to the brain of oxygen, nutrients or hormones. Dementia is not a single disease, but a term used to encompass a variety of brain diseases. The most common causes of dementia in the elderly are Alzheimer's disease and multi-infarct dementia (recurrent mini-strokes of cortical/subcortical areas).

Confusion is where an individual has difficulty placing herself in terms of time and/or place. It can lead to disorientation, loss of short-term memory, changed levels of activity, speech defects, hallucinations and clouding of consciousness. Acute confusion (delirium) is a relatively common finding amongst elderly people. It may also be an important indicator of an underlying systemic disease (e.g. CVA, infection). Confusion may be aggravated by drugs (e.g. alcohol), sight or hearing defects and presence of other brain diseases (e.g. Parkinson's disease). Confusion may also be a feature of acute or chronic dementia.

**Table 18.10** Mental test score

1. Name
2. Date of birth
3. Age
4. Date and time of day
5. Address
6. Name of prime minister
7. Date of First World War
8. Place
9. Remember an address 5 min later
10. Count backwards from 20 to 1

Assessment of mental state can easily be achieved by means of a mental test score (Table 18.10). This is performed by the practitioner asking 10 simple questions to the patient. A low score (less than 7) indicates confusion and warrants referral to other agencies (e.g. GP, psychiatrist). Deterioration in mental test score may indicate the presence of a chronic dementing illness (e.g. Alzheimer's disease).

## Assessment of ability to perform basic foot care

For the practitioner, accurate determination of an elderly patient's ability to perform basic tasks relating to foot care will be important. The following activities are important as part of personal activities of daily living:

- cutting and/or filing of toe nails
- filing of hard skin
- application of cream to the sole of the foot
- washing and drying of feet
- putting on stockings, tights or socks
- putting on and fastening shoes
- change of a dressing applied to the foot (where appropriate)
- inspection of feet for lesions.

Inability to perform the above activities may place an elderly person at greater risk of deteriorating foot health. This is particularly likely where the elderly person is not able (or eligible) to receive podiatric care and where there is an assumption that the person will manage her own feet. Failure to perform these basic activities may ultimately also contribute to deterioration in mobility, independence and quality of life. For example, patients may feel less inclined to go outside of the house if putting on shoes and hosiery becomes difficult. Provision of simple aids, such as elasticated laces and stocking helpers, can sometimes rectify this problem, by providing assistance with difficult activities.

Inability to check and clean feet can be a major risk for deterioration in foot health status. This is especially true for patients with either peripheral vascular insufficiency or defects of sensory perception. Sight defects may compound the problem. In these cases, the patient should be encouraged to ask a carer to check their feet regularly, or seek regular professional assessment.

The best way to assess an individual's ability to perform basic foot care tasks is to observe them being performed. Practitioners should spend some time with patients looking for signs of difficulty reaching feet, putting on shoes and hosiery, and problems with manual dexterity (e.g. arthritis of fingers). This can often be determined during the course of a normal consultation:

- Is the patient able to take off and put back on her own shoes and hosiery?
- Can the patient touch areas of her feet?
- Is the patient able to manipulate a pair of scissors/nippers?
- Can the patient manage the use of a file?
- Can the patient apply a cream to the foot?
- Is the patient able to change a dressing on her foot?

It is important for the practitioner observing these skills to bear in mind that conditions in the patient's own home may be totally different to those in the clinical environment. Patients may find it easy to manage their feet while seated in a podiatry chair, but find the same tasks difficult in an armchair or on a sofa or bed.

## RISK ASSESSMENT AND THE ELDERLY

Limited resources for public podiatry services have resulted in attempts to prioritise services to those people most at risk. Usually, notions of risk have centred on medical need for foot care. It is clearly a worthy desire to focus limited resources on those most at need. However, risk assessment of the elderly can be a hazardous pursuit and should not be undertaken without appropriate validation of risk assessment protocols.

The risks of prioritisation are enormous, both to individuals and to health services. Getting it wrong has major consequences for individuals (ulceration, infection, falls, gangrene, amputation) and for health services (litigation, complaints, costs of managing complications, effect on other service providers, etc.).

Generally, the elderly can be divided into three groups in respect of risk status: high risk, medium risk and low risk (Table 18.11). What

**Table 18.11** Definitions of elderly risk groups

| | |
|---|---|
| High risk | Patients with systemic pathology presenting a risk to foot health (e.g. diabetes mellitus, Cushing's disease, leukaemia, anaemia, etc.) Patients with existing foot ulceration or other loss of lower limb tissue viability Patients who have a history of falls Patients with peripheral vascular disease Patients with peripheral neuropathy Patients with hip joint pathology or prosthesis Patients who are bed-ridden Malnourished patients Patients taking certain medications (steroids, anticoagulants, anticancer drugs, etc.) Patients with severe cognitive impairment Patients unable to self-care with poor carer support Infirm or frail people living alone Poor patients Socially isolated patients |
| Medium risk | Patients with poor skin quality or skin disease Patients with thickened nails Patients with calluses or corns Patients with toe deformities Immobile patients Patients with superficial fungal infections of skin or nail Patients unable to self-care with adequate carer support |
| Low risk | Patients with mild foot pathology Patients with good circulatory status Patients with good neurological status Independent patients or those receiving good levels of home care Mobile patients Patients with good personal care/hygiene |

becomes clear when looking at these definitions is that most podiatry departments are already focusing on those at greatest risk.

Several providers of foot health services have attempted to use risk 'scoring' methods to make decisions on eligibility for podiatry services. These criteria are often rigidly applied, allow no professional discretion and are sometimes administered by people other than those specialised in the assessment of the lower limb. Where risk assessment protocols are used, it is important for practitioners using such protocols to be able to obtain second opinions, and identify patients who they feel are at risk but who do not fit the 'rigid' criteria.

Risk assessment of the elderly is further complicated by the fact that elderly people tend to deteriorate much faster than young people. An elderly person who seems quite fit today may be infirm or ill tomorrow. This effect can have devastating consequences for foot health where a patient is under the impression that they are no longer eligible for foot care.

Reassessment of the elderly patient is necessary at regular intervals. Risk status changes with corresponding changes in general health status, physiological changes and social circumstances. Even changes in time of the year can have a profound effect on risk status. For example, during the summer a patient may appear to have adequate peripheral circulation, but the same patient might assess as high risk during the winter when circulation deteriorates.

The most effective risk assessment protocols have used qualitative descriptors of risk rather than rigid/quantitative risk-scoring mechanisms. Effective risk assessment is dependent upon the following:

- existence of a valid risk assessment protocol
- patient understanding of the process
- compliance of the patient with advice
- availability and motivation of carers (where appropriate)
- awareness of GPs (and others) of the protocols/eligibility for re-referral
- ability to reassess/review risk status as required.

Even the most effective risk assessment protocol fails from time to time and patients who were identified as low risk may develop serious pathology. Where risk assessment does fail, departments need to ensure that patients can receive rapid assessment and treatment to prevent the likelihood of significant adverse consequences.

It is impossible to be completely certain when assessing the risk of individuals, particularly the old. Health providers need to weigh up the costs (personal, social and economic) of risk assessment with the costs of universal provision of podiatry services.

## SUMMARY

This chapter has examined a range of factors that are pertinent to the assessment of the elderly. Although the overall assessment process for the elderly should be no different to that of any other age group there are specific factors that should be taken into consideration. It is essential that practitioners are aware that any assessment of the elderly provides a snap shot of the elderly person at the time of the assessment. In view of the ageing process and increased risk of acquiring a range of diseases the status of the elderly person may change from low to high risk within a relatively short period of time.

REFERENCES

Bennett G C J, Ebrahim S 1995 health care in old age, 2nd edn. Arnold, London
Clearing House's web site: (http://www.leeds.ac.uk/nuffield/infoservices/UKCH/home.html)
Crawford V L S, Ashford R L, McPeake B, Stout R W 1995 Conservative podiatric medicine and disability in elderly people. Journal of the American Podiatric Medical Association 85(5): 255–259
Hansard 1998. HMSO, London
Harvey I, Frankel S, Marks R, Shalom D, Morgan M 1997 Foot morbidity and exposure to chiropody: population based study. British Medical Journal 315: 1054–1055

body. Because surgical techniques require their use, any contraindication to local anaesthetics must be identified. The following contraindications should be considered:

**Unstable epilepsy.** High blood levels of local anaesthetic agents are known to cause convulsions in some epileptic patients through their action on brain tissue. Their use is therefore best avoided in such individuals.

**Methaemoglobinaemia.** Methaemoglobin is a form of haemoglobin consisting of globin with an oxidised haem-containing ferric iron. Methaemoglobin is unable to transport oxygen and therefore compromises cardiovascular function. When prilocaine is metabolised by the liver, small amounts of a chemical called 0-toluidine are produced which inhibits the enzyme involved in the conversion of methaemoglobin to haemoglobin. In patients with known methaemoglobinaemia, an alternative local anaesthetic agent to prilocaine should be utilised.

**Pregnancy and breastfeeding.** The British Medical Association suggests that drugs should only be used during pregnancy where the potential benefit outweighs the risk of harm to the fetus, particularly during the first trimester where all drugs should be avoided if possible. There is no specific guidance on the risks associated with the low doses of local anaesthesia used in the foot of a pregnant woman. However, because of the ability of local anaesthetics to cross the placental barrier, they are probably best avoided whenever possible during pregnancy. If a local anaesthetic were to be given during pregnancy it would seem prudent to avoid prilocaine hydrochloride, as fetal haemoglobin is more susceptible to the development of methaemoglobinaemia. Both lidocaine (lignocaine) and bupivacaine are considered safe for use with breastfeeding mothers, as the quantities secreted into breast milk are small.

**Porphyrias.** The porphyrias are a group of metabolic disorders. Included in the list of drugs contraindicated for use in patients with porphyria are some local anaesthetics. These drugs must therefore be avoided in known carriers of the porphyrogenic gene to avoid precipitating an acute attack.

Where surgery is still indicated, the use of a general anaesthetic should be considered and the patient referred.

### Psychiatric status

Patients approach surgery with an understandable amount of fear and anxiety. They know that they will be in an unfamiliar environment to which they are unaccustomed. Some fear that they will experience pain during the operation. Most of their anxiety is down to inadequate knowledge based on hearsay and rumour.

During the preoperative assessment it is important that the practitioner recognises the hypernervous patient and provides appropriate information and counselling to allay any concerns. However, it is important that the practitioner recognises when a patient is unsuitable for surgery under local anaesthesia and, if surgery is necessary, refers the patient for general anaesthesia.

### Age

**Older patients.** An increasing percentage of the population is over 65 years of age, a trend that is expected to continue well into the 21st century. Independent ambulation is an important component of wellness, although a majority of patients over the age of 65 complain of foot pain limiting their activity. In geriatric patients who have foot conditions which can be surgically corrected, and where the physical condition is satisfactory, surgery can safely be performed. The chronological age of the patient is less important, as long as the physiological age of the patient is adequate for the planned surgical procedure.

The problems of surgery on the older patient include:

- an adverse physiological status
- impact of surgery on the patient's lifestyle
- selection of the operative procedure – simple procedures versus complex procedures – even though the latter would give a better result.

Generally, in the older patient, it is found that destructive rather than functionally reconstructive procedures are often more appropriate.

**Children.** Attention to the child's psychology, patient–parent relationships and stress levels is important in the surgical treatment of the paediatric patient. Parental presence during the operation may be beneficial.

### Infection

In general, the elective procedure is performed when the patient is free from all systemic infection. A patient with established infection that does not respond to oral antibiotics and appropriate wound care demands a thorough preoperative evaluation and specialty consultation.

## Laboratory investigations and imaging modalities

**Urine testing.** As indicated in Chapter 13, urinalysis is an aid in the diagnosis of renal disease, hepatic disease and diabetes mellitus. Diabetes mellitus can have widespread consequences for the lower limb and is of particular interest to the surgeon. Renal and hepatic diseases may have serious systemic repercussions and, if identified, require further investigation before it is safe to proceed with surgery. Urinalysis is therefore useful in the preoperative assessment of patients to screen for illnesses which may complicate or contraindicate elective procedures. Screening for a urinary tract infection (UTI) or the presence of bacteria in urine can also identify those patients at increased risk of developing postoperative wound infections. Testing is non-invasive and cost-effective, and urine specimens are easily obtained.

**Blood analysis.** The use of blood analysis in the preoperative assessment of the surgical patient is a matter for debate. Routine screening prior to surgery is likely to reveal a small percentage of abnormality, most of which is insignificant to anaesthetic or surgical management in any case. Therefore, the general rule for the use of confirmatory diagnostic testing should apply: their use is indicated from the initial patient assessment. In cases where systemic pathology is known or suspected – e.g. in anaemia to ascertain haemoglobin levels – blood sampling is most certainly indicated.

The patient on anticoagulant therapy has already been discussed. Similarly, patients who suffer from clotting abnormalities also require further investigation (Table 19.5).

**Radiographs.** Radiographs are vital to the surgeon for a number of reasons:

- they allow the identification of many rheumatological, metabolic, endocrine and infective disease states
- they allow the progression of deformity to be monitored
- they show the precise relationship between osseous anatomical structures that are of particular interest to the surgeon
- they aid in the selection of the most appropriate surgical technique
- they demonstrate the position of retained internal fixation and are used to confirm bone healing in the postoperative phase.

The identification and use of angular relationships, or charting, between the foot bones has become a key skill of the podiatrist.

Osteoporosis begins in middle life and is predominantly a disease of postmenopausal women. Histologically, bone formation is normal, but bone resorption is increased. If preoperative radiographs suggest significant osteoporosis, systemic disease is likely and multiple contributing factors, including dietary deficiencies, endocrine imbalances, sedentary lifestyles and genetic predisposition, may be implicated. The implications for the fixation of osteotomies are clear. Radiographic assessment is covered in Chapter 11.

**Table 19.5** Common clotting abnormalities

von Willebrand's disease
Haemophilia
    Type A – classical haemophilia
    Type B – Christmas disease
    Type C – PTA (plasma thromboplastin antecedent)
        deficiency
Vitamin K deficiency